PRACTICAL APPROACHES TO CLINICAL DIAGNOSIS

PRACTICAL APPROACHES TO CLINICAL DIAGNOSIS

A STEP-BY-STEP GUIDE TO DIAGNOSIS

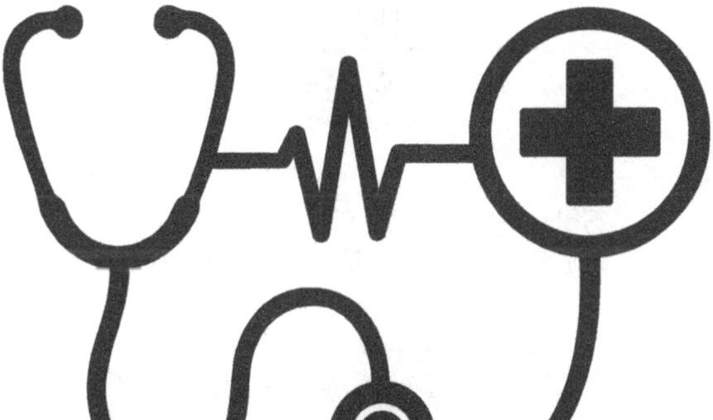

DR OMAR HASSOUNA

BROWN DOG BOOKS

First published 2026

Published under licence by Brown Dog Books and
The Self-Publishing Partnership Ltd, 10b Greenway Farm, Bath Rd,
Wick, nr. Bath BS30 5RL, UK

ISBN printed book: 978-1-918428-19-3
ISBN e-book: 978-1-918428-20-9

Cover design by Kevin Rylands
Internal design by Mac Style

Printed and bound in the UK

This book is printed on FSC® certified paper

MIX
Paper | Supporting responsible forestry
FSC® C013604

To my wife and children, whose love, patience, and support carried me through this journey.

Contents

Introduction

Clinical practice today is increasingly constrained by time, complexity, and cost. Clinicians are required to reach accurate diagnoses efficiently while avoiding unnecessary investigation and delay. This book was written to address that challenge.

Practical Approaches to Clinical Diagnosis focuses on structured, real-world clinical reasoning rather than exhaustive detail. It is intended for medical students, junior doctors, general practitioners, and other frontline clinicians who regularly assess undifferentiated symptoms. The emphasis throughout is on recognising common patterns, identifying danger signals early, and investigating logically.

By encouraging disciplined thinking, careful history-taking, and selective use of investigations, this book aims to save time, reduce unnecessary referrals and testing, and support safer, more cost-effective patient care. In doing so, it seeks to benefit both patients and the wider healthcare system, including the NHS.

"This book starts where the patient starts —
not where the textbook starts."

Topic 1

Anaemia

Note: this topic has been presented in detail because of its clinical breadth and the importance of structured diagnostic reasoning in everyday practice.

Anaemia is a frequent finding in primary care, affecting all age groups and clinical settings. It presents with a wide spectrum of underlying causes. In many cases, diagnosis is straightforward with a full blood count and peripheral blood film, yet in others it remains complex and demands a structured, stepwise approach. The challenge is twofold: first, to confirm and classify anaemia, and second, to identify the underlying cause. A systematic strategy saves time and resources while ensuring patient safety.

Anaemia typically manifests with fatigue, exertional breathlessness, and generalised tiredness, all reflecting reduced oxygen delivery to the tissues. The severity of symptoms depends not only on the haemoglobin level but also on age, comorbidities, occupational demands, and the rapidity of onset. In elderly patients or those with ischaemic heart disease or heart failure, even mild anaemia can worsen the underlying condition, precipitating angina or decompensation.

In severe cases, particularly among older individuals, cognitive decline or confusion may be the initial complaint. Physical signs may include pallor of the skin, conjunctivae, or nail beds, though this may be absent even in severe anaemia. Some patients develop evidence of high-output cardiac failure, such as tachycardia, a soft ejection systolic murmur, and ankle oedema.

The first step is to confirm anaemia with a full blood count. Once confirmed, the red-cell indices and blood film guide classification. Anaemia is broadly divided into three patterns: microcytic, normocytic, and macrocytic, and this framework provides the foundation for further investigation. Microcytic anaemia is characterised by a reduced mean corpuscular volume and, usually, a low mean corpuscular haemoglobin concentration.

The most common cause worldwide is iron deficiency, which may result from chronic gastrointestinal blood loss, menorrhagia, poor dietary intake, or malabsorption. Inflammatory conditions and malignancy may cause functional iron deficiency, in which iron is sequestered and unavailable for haemoglobin production.

Less frequent causes include sideroblastic anaemia, in which iron cannot be effectively incorporated into haemoglobin, and the thalassaemias and related haemoglobinopathies, which are inherited disorders of globin chain synthesis. Investigations are directed by clinical suspicion. Iron studies are essential to assess stores and utilisation, and if gastrointestinal blood loss is suspected, endoscopic assessment may be required. In regions or populations where thalassaemia or sickle cell disease is more prevalent, haemoglobin electrophoresis can be invaluable.

Normocytic anaemia often presents a diagnostic challenge because of the wide range of possible causes. Acute or chronic blood loss may lead to this pattern, as may anaemia of chronic disease, which accompanies conditions such as tuberculosis, rheumatoid arthritis, or malignancy. Bone marrow disorders, including multiple myeloma and other myeloproliferative diseases, may also present with this pattern. Chronic kidney disease leads to reduced erythropoietin production, while endocrine disorders such as hypothyroidism and Addison's disease can suppress red cell production.

Haemolytic anaemia, whether autoimmune or non-immune in origin, represents another important category. Investigations again depend on context. Renal function tests are essential when kidney disease is suspected. Inflammatory markers and autoimmune screening can help identify systemic disease, while serum protein electrophoresis is useful in evaluating suspected myeloma. The reticulocyte count provides an indication of bone marrow response, and in complex or unclear cases, bone marrow biopsy may be required.

Macrocytic anaemia is defined by an elevated mean corpuscular volume and the presence of abnormal red-cell morphology. The most common causes include vitamin B12 deficiency, often due to pernicious anaemia, dietary insufficiency, malabsorption, or previous gastrectomy, and folate deficiency, which is frequently related to poor diet, alcoholism, malabsorption, or pregnancy.

Chronic alcohol intake and liver disease also contribute, while hypothyroidism may be a less obvious cause. Bone marrow disorders such as myelodysplastic syndromes and certain medications, particularly methotrexate, complete the list of major considerations. Investigations should include measurements of vitamin B12 and folate, along with thyroid and liver function tests. Where there is uncertainty, bone marrow examination may be required.

In daily general practice, however, the vast majority of cases fall into predictable patterns. Microcytic anaemia is most often due to iron deficiency. The main causes of this deficiency are menstrual blood loss in women, microscopic gastrointestinal bleeding such as from peptic ulcer or malignancy, and, less frequently, poor diet or malabsorption. Normocytic anaemia is usually secondary to chronic disease, reflecting an underlying process such as chronic renal failure, long-standing rheumatological or inflammatory disorders, or malignant disease. In such cases, red-cell production is suppressed despite adequate iron stores. Macrocytic anaemia, on the other hand, most commonly results from vitamin B12 or folate deficiency. This may be related to autoimmune gastritis, previous gastric or ileal surgery, malabsorption syndromes, or excessive alcohol intake. In many patients with chronic alcohol use or liver disease, macrocytosis may occur even in the absence of overt anaemia.

The sheer number of possible causes can make anaemia appear daunting, but the clinician should always adopt a pragmatic, stepwise strategy. The starting point is classification into microcytic, normocytic, or macrocytic categories. From there, the key question becomes: what is the most common cause in this patient? In primary care, iron deficiency is by far the most frequent and should always be considered first. Investigations should proceed sequentially, focusing on the most probable explanation and reserving rarer diagnoses for later consideration. This reflects real-world reasoning – efficient, logical, and resource-conscious. For example, in a 40-year-old woman with heavy menstrual bleeding, iron deficiency is far more likely than myelodysplasia, and investigating bone marrow disease first would waste resources and generate unnecessary anxiety.

Anaemia is both common and multifaceted. Recognition often begins with a routine blood test, yet the underlying cause may range from simple iron deficiency to serious marrow pathology. A structured approach ensures timely and cost-effective diagnosis. The clinician should first confirm anaemia, then classify it, and finally investigate the most likely causes in a logical order. This method saves time, avoids unnecessary testing, and ensures that serious conditions are not overlooked. Ultimately, efficient diagnosis of anaemia improves patient outcomes while safeguarding healthcare resources.

Topic 2

Haematuria

Haematuria, or blood in the urine, is a common but could be a serious finding and a symptom of an underlying condition. The first step is to confirm that it is truly blood. A dipstick test alone is unreliable because it reacts with haemoglobin and myoglobin as well as red blood cells. Urine microscopy is therefore essential. If red cells are seen, haematuria is confirmed. If none are present, consider haemoglobinuria or myoglobinuria. Drugs such as rifampicin, some food dyes, and beetroot can also discolour urine and should be excluded before further investigation. Early and accurate confirmation saves both time and unnecessary anxiety for the patient.

Once true blood is confirmed, causes can be grouped as renal, urinary, or systemic.

Renal causes include glomerulonephritis, renal stones, pyelonephritis, and renal tumours.

Urinary tract causes are more frequent and include bladder cancer, cystitis, trauma, radiation cystitis, and urethritis. In men, the prostate is a common source through benign enlargement, infection, or carcinoma.

Systemic causes include anticoagulant use, bleeding disorders, and severe hypertension. In women, contamination from menstruation should always be considered, particularly when the urine sample is not obtained midstream.

Symptoms vary according to the source of bleeding. Painless visible haematuria in adults is particularly concerning and must always be investigated for malignancy. Painful haematuria with dysuria or frequency suggests infection. Colicky flank pain indicates stones. Hesitancy, poor stream, or nocturia point to prostatic enlargement. Fever, rigors, or malaise imply infection, while oedema or frothy urine may indicate renal involvement. Weight loss, fatigue, or bone pain should always raise concern about malignancy.

Examination should be focused and brief. Assess general condition and blood pressure carefully, as hypertension may accompany renal disease. Look for pallor or oedema. Examine the abdomen and flanks for tenderness or masses, and palpate the bladder for distension. Suprapubic tenderness suggests cystitis; loin tenderness points to stones or pyelonephritis. In men, a rectal examination is required to assess the prostate, while in women a pelvic examination may be appropriate when local causes are suspected.

Investigations should be purposeful and guided by the clinical picture. Confirm red cells with microscopy and send urine for culture and sensitivity. Check renal function, full blood count, and, if necessary, a coagulation profile. Ultrasound of the kidneys and bladder is the best first-line imaging to identify stones, obstruction, or masses. Cystoscopy is indicated for visible haematuria or unexplained microscopic haematuria, especially in patients over forty or with risk factors such as smoking or occupational chemical exposure. CT urography is reserved for upper-tract assessment when malignancy or stones are suspected. Every investigation must have a clear reason; unnecessary testing wastes both time and resources.

Because the range of causes is wide, the clinician must focus on the common and clinically significant ones. In practice, most cases of haematuria arise from four main causes forming the essential diagnostic block:

1. Urinary tract infection
2. Renal or ureteric stones
3. Benign prostatic enlargement
4. Urinary tract malignancy

These four conditions account for the majority of presentations in both primary and secondary care. Concentrating on them allows the clinician to investigate efficiently, avoiding confusion and delay.

Urinary tract infection is the commonest cause and is usually accompanied by dysuria, frequency, and urgency.

Renal or ureteric stones cause sharp flank pain radiating to the groin, sometimes with visible blood.

Benign prostatic enlargement occurs mainly in older men and may cause intermittent bleeding with obstructive symptoms.

Urinary tract malignancy, particularly bladder cancer, often presents as painless visible haematuria and must always be excluded.

Once these four have been considered and appropriate investigations performed, attention may then shift to less frequent causes only when necessary.

A clear and disciplined approach prevents confusion. Confirm the presence of true blood, take a concise history, perform a directed examination, and test logically for these four common causes first. Only after excluding them should rarer systemic or renal conditions be explored. This logical sequence saves time, reduces cost, and maintains high standards of patient care.

For the general practitioner, the priorities are early recognition, initial assessment, and prompt referral when indicated. For hospital doctors, the emphasis is on structured reasoning and accurate diagnosis without unnecessary repetition. Clear communication between primary and secondary care ensures continuity and safe follow-up for the patient.

Haematuria should never be regarded as trivial. Even when infection or stones appear likely, malignancy must remain under consideration until excluded. A logical and cost-effective diagnostic approach ensures that significant disease is recognised early and that patients receive appropriate and timely treatment.

The message is clear: confirm that blood is present, focus on the four principal causes - urinary tract infection, renal or ureteric stones, benign prostatic enlargement, and malignancy - and investigate with purpose. This approach is cost-effective, time-saving, and clinically sound, ensuring rapid and safe patient care.

Topic 3

Back Pain

Back pain is one of the commonest complaints in both primary and secondary care. It contributes greatly to morbidity, loss of work, and the economic burden on society. Almost every adult will experience back pain at some point, and for many it becomes a recurring problem.

Because of its frequency, clinicians may underestimate its potential seriousness, yet missing important pathology carries clinical and medico-legal consequences. For this reason, the subject demands a clear diagnostic framework that is simple, time-efficient, and cost-effective.

For practical purposes, back pain is best divided into three broad groups. The first is mechanical pain, by far the most common. The second is non-mechanical pain, which includes inflammatory, infective, osteoporotic, and malignant causes. The third is visceral pain, in which disease within the abdomen or retroperitoneum is perceived as pain in the back. These categories provide a foundation to structure the consultation and prevent diagnostic distraction.

Mechanical causes dominate. Simple muscle or ligament strain is the usual culprit, often related to lifting, awkward movement, or prolonged poor posture. These patients present with localised lumbar pain - sometimes sharp, sometimes aching - worsened by activity and eased by rest or gentle movement.

Disc prolapse may produce nerve-root irritation with pain radiating down one leg in the classic pattern of sciatica. In older adults, spinal stenosis caused by degenerative narrowing can present with neurogenic claudication. Degenerative arthritis of the spine, or spondylosis, is also very common. Structural deformities such as scoliosis or kyphosis may contribute, especially if longstanding.

Non-mechanical causes, though less frequent, are more serious. Infection may appear as discitis, vertebral osteomyelitis, or spinal tuberculosis. Inflammatory disease such as ankylosing spondylitis typically affects younger adults and produces prolonged morning stiffness that improves with exercise.

Osteoporosis predisposes to compression fractures, especially in elderly patients and in those taking corticosteroids. Malignancy, whether primary or metastatic, must always be borne in mind, particularly in patients with a relevant past history or systemic symptoms.

Visceral causes complete the picture. The kidneys, pancreas, and aorta are the principal organs whose disorders can manifest as back pain. Renal colic produces severe, fluctuating pain radiating from the loin to the groin. Pancreatitis causes intense epigastric pain that bores through to the back. An abdominal aortic aneurysm may present with sudden or persistent back pain, sometimes pulsatile, and represents a medical emergency.

Clinical features vary with the underlying cause. Mechanical pain is often localised to the lumbar area, aggravated by specific movements, and may be accompanied by muscle spasm. Disc-related pain radiates in a dermatomal pattern, while spinal stenosis causes leg pain on walking that settles with rest.

Inflammatory pain is recognised by morning stiffness and nocturnal discomfort. Infective or malignant pain tends to persist at rest and may be associated with fever or weight loss. Visceral pain is often atypical in site or character and may be accompanied by abdominal or systemic features.

Examination must be systematic yet efficient. Observation of posture and gait provides immediate clues. Palpation may reveal paraspinal tenderness or, more importantly, focal bony tenderness suggesting fracture, infection, or tumour.

Spinal movement is restricted in proportion to pain in mechanical cases, but remains limited even at rest in inflammatory or structural disease.

Neurological examination of the lower limbs is essential. Power, reflexes, and sensation should be checked to detect nerve-root compromise.

A positive straight-leg raise may indicate disc irritation, but definite weakness, sensory loss, or reflex asymmetry provide stronger evidence of compression. Perineal sensation must be assessed if cauda equina syndrome is suspected.

Investigations are chosen according to context. In typical acute mechanical back pain without warning signs, no investigation is required initially. Where infection, inflammation, or malignancy is suspected, blood tests such as full blood count, ESR, and CRP are helpful.

Urinalysis may assist in identifying renal or urinary causes. Plain spinal X-rays have limited value in acute cases, but can reveal fractures, deformities, or severe degenerative change. Magnetic resonance imaging is the investigation of choice when neurological deficit, disc prolapse, infection, or malignancy is suspected.

Computed tomography is useful for detailed bony assessment or when MRI is contraindicated. The key principle is that every investigation must have a defined diagnostic purpose.

With so many possibilities, the clinician must maintain a clear diagnostic block. The first question is always whether the pain is mechanical. In the vast majority of primary-care patients, it is, and a careful history and examination usually confirm this.

The next question is whether any red flags are present. These include constant pain at rest or nocturnal pain; neurological compromise, in patients with marked thirst such as foot drop or bladder and bowel disturbance; and systemic symptoms such as fever, weight loss, or a history of cancer. If any of these are identified, urgent investigation and referral are required.

Only after common mechanical causes and red flags have been addressed should attention shift to the less common inflammatory, infective, or malignant conditions. These are far less frequent in general practice, but must be recognised because of their severity.

Finally, rare causes – such as unusual tumours or metabolic bone disease – should be considered only when all other explanations fail. Proceeding in this order avoids wasted time and unnecessary tests, while remaining alert to serious disease.

One further point deserves emphasis. Back pain is not only a clinical challenge but also a medico-legal risk. The conditions most often missed – and most commonly leading to litigation – are cauda equina syndrome, metastatic disease, and spinal infection.

Failure to recognise bladder or bowel disturbance, saddle anaesthesia, or rapidly progressive neurological deficit can result in permanent disability. Ignoring systemic signs which suggest cancer or infection also endangers both patient and doctor. Accurate documentation of history, red-flag screening, examination findings, and reasoning for investigation is therefore essential.

In summary, back pain is extremely common and its causes are many. The safe and efficient diagnostic approach is to classify broadly into mechanical, non-mechanical, and visceral; to use history and examination to confirm the common mechanical diagnosis first; to identify red flags early; and only then to consider the less common and rare causes.

Following this structured sequence saves time, conserves resources, and ensures safe and effective patient care while minimising the risk of missed diagnosis or legal repercussions.

The message is clear: recognise mechanical causes early, search for red flags diligently, and investigate with purpose. This approach is cost-effective, time-saving, and clinically safe.

Topic 4

Jaundice

Jaundice is a common clinical sign encountered in practice. Although it is not seen every day in general practice, every doctor will face it at some point, and it can reflect anything from mild self-limiting illness to severe life-threatening disease. Because of this wide spectrum, the clinician must follow a structured diagnostic approach that saves time, preserves resources, and ensures patient safety.

For practical purposes, jaundice is classified into three categories: pre-hepatic, hepatic, and post-hepatic. This classification is useful because it reflects where in the bilirubin pathway the disturbance occurs.

Pre-hepatic jaundice, also known as haemolytic jaundice, arises from increased bilirubin production due to red cell breakdown or ineffective erythropoiesis. The liver itself functions normally, conjugating bilirubin, but unconjugated bilirubin accumulates in the blood. Common causes include sickle cell anaemia, thalassaemia, G6PD deficiency, hereditary spherocytosis, autoimmune haemolysis, and infections such as malaria or sepsis. Drug-induced haemolysis and large haematomas are additional contributors. Because unconjugated bilirubin is not water soluble, it does not appear in the urine, which remains normal in colour.

Hepatic jaundice occurs when the liver's function is impaired, so bilirubin is only partially conjugated. The unconjugated fraction remains in the blood and is not excreted in urine .Causes include acute viral hepatitis, drug-induced hepatitis (for example from paracetamol or isoniazid), and chronic liver disease such as cirrhosis, whether due to alcohol or non-alcoholic fatty liver disease. Genetic disorders like Dubin-Johnson syndrome and Crigler-

Najjar syndrome, though rare, are recognised causes. Certain infections, including leptospirosis and yellow fever, may also lead to hepatic jaundice.

Post-hepatic jaundice, or obstructive jaundice, develops when conjugated bilirubin cannot pass freely through the biliary system and instead refluxes into the blood. As conjugated bilirubin is water soluble, it is excreted in the urine, giving it a dark, tea-coloured appearance. Common causes include gallstones in the common bile duct, carcinoma of the pancreas, cholangiocarcinoma, and biliary strictures or cholangitis. Clinically, patients often present with deep jaundice, pruritus, pale stools, and dark urine.

A detailed history is crucial. The age of the patient immediately helps narrow the differential. In younger patients, acute viral hepatitis, drug-induced hepatitis, or inherited haemolytic disorders are more likely. In older patients, especially those with significant weight loss and itching, an obstructive cause such as carcinoma of the pancreas or gallstones in the common bile duct is more probable. Additional history should cover alcohol intake, drug exposure, blood transfusions, travel, and family history of haemoglobinopathies or hereditary liver disease.

Symptoms provide strong clues. Deep jaundice with pruritus and weight loss, particularly in an elderly patient, points towards obstruction. Fever and malaise following drug exposure suggest hepatic involvement. A history of recurrent anaemia or haemolytic crisis in a younger person suggests pre-hepatic jaundice. The colour of urine and stool is often diagnostic: dark urine and pale stools strongly indicate obstruction, whereas normal urine colour is more consistent with haemolysis.

Examination follows naturally from the history. Look for stigmata of chronic liver disease such as spider naevl, palmar erythema, ascites, hepatomegaly, or splenomegaly. Ankle oedema and flapping tremor may suggest advanced hepatic failure. A palpable gallbladder in a jaundiced patient raises the suspicion of malignant obstruction (Courvoisier's sign). General examination may reveal anaemia in haemolysis or lymphadenopathy in malignancy or infection.

Investigations should be ordered with purpose. Liver function tests help distinguish hepatocellular injury from cholestasis: raised transaminases suggest hepatic disease, while elevated alkaline phosphatase and conjugated bilirubin suggest obstruction. A full blood count may show anaemia in haemolysis, and a raised reticulocyte count supports the diagnosis. Viral serology and autoimmune markers may be needed in hepatic cases.

Urinalysis revealing dark urine provides a quick clue to conjugated hyperbilirubinaemia. Imaging is indispensable: ultrasound is the first-line tool to detect gallstones, biliary dilatation, or pancreatic masses. Where more detail is needed, CT or MRCP can provide further information.

At this stage the clinician may feel overwhelmed by the wide differential, but the solution is to build a diagnostic block. The first question should always be: what are the most common causes in this clinical context? In everyday practice, obstructive jaundice from gallstones or pancreatic malignancy is a leading cause in older adults, while viral hepatitis or drug-induced hepatitis dominate in the young. Haemolytic causes are less frequent in general practice but must not be overlooked, particularly in populations with haemoglobinopathies or malaria.

The second question is: what is most dangerous? Severe obstructive jaundice, acute fulminant hepatitis, and rapidly progressive liver failure are all emergencies. Red flags include deep jaundice with systemic deterioration, encephalopathy, or unexplained weight loss in an elderly patient. These must be recognised without delay.

Once the common and dangerous causes have been considered, the uncommon and rare can be explored. These include hereditary conditions such as Dubin–Johnson or Crigler–Najjar syndrome, or unusual infections such as leptospirosis. Considering them only after the common and dangerous ensures efficiency and prevents wasted resources.

Finally, the medico-legal dimension cannot be ignored. Misdiagnosis or delayed recognition of obstructive jaundice, particularly due to carcinoma of the pancreas, is a frequent source of litigation. Similarly, failure to identify fulminant hepatitis or jaundice associated with sepsis or haemolysis can have grave consequences. Protection lies in a systematic approach: documenting a thorough history, screening for red flags, recording examination findings, explaining the reasoning behind investigations, and giving patients clear guidance about when to return. Good communication and precise notes safeguard both patient and clinician.

In summary, jaundice has a wide range of causes, but the diagnostic approach can be simplified. Classify into pre-hepatic, hepatic, and post-hepatic. Take a careful history, guided by age and associated features. Examine systematically for signs that point to liver, blood, or biliary disease. Use targeted investigations to confirm the likely diagnosis. Above all, focus first on the common causes, remain alert for the dangerous ones, and move to the uncommon and rare only when the basics have been excluded. This structured method saves time, conserves resources, and ensures safe, effective care.

Topic 5

Polyuria

Polyuria is defined as an abnormally high volume of urine output, usually more than three litres per day in an adult. It is important to distinguish this from urinary frequency, where the patient passes small amounts often, but without an increased daily total. Many patients confuse the two, and clarifying the difference at the outset avoids unnecessary investigations and directs the clinician towards the right causes.

Patients with true polyuria may present in different settings. Some arrive in the emergency department with acute dehydration or metabolic imbalance. Others are referred to outpatient clinics for unexplained excessive urine output. However, most commonly, polyuria is first raised in primary care. A general practitioner may be told by a patient that they 'cannot stop going to the toilet,' or that they are 'up all night passing water.' Such complaints can generate anxiety, particularly if the patient suspects kidney disease or diabetes. For the GP, the task is to establish whether polyuria is genuine, identify the likely cause, and decide whether simple tests will suffice or whether referral is required.

In everyday practice, three causes dominate. Diabetes mellitus is the leading explanation. Once plasma glucose rises above the renal threshold, glucose appears in the urine. Being osmotically active, it drags water with it, producing a large volume of urine. Patients often report excessive thirst, nocturia, blurred vision, recurrent infections, or weight loss. Sometimes, polyuria is the very symptom that leads to the discovery of previously undiagnosed diabetes. For this reason, glucose testing is the first and most essential step when a patient presents with polyuria.

Drug-induced polyuria is also common. Diuretics are widely prescribed for hypertension and heart failure, and they predictably increase urine output. For most patients this is expected, but some may find the effect troublesome. In recent years, SGLT2 inhibitors such as dapagliflozin have become increasingly used. These promote glycosuria, leading to a mild osmotic diuresis. Although this is a therapeutic effect, many patients interpret it as abnormal, and reassurance from the GP is often all that is needed.

The third major cause is hypercalcaemia. Excess calcium interferes with the kidney's ability to concentrate urine, leading to water loss and polyuria. Depending on the underlying condition, patients may also complain of constipation, abdominal pain, fatigue, or bone pain. Hypercalcaemia is most often due to primary hyperparathyroidism or malignancy, but whatever the cause, polyuria is frequently the symptom that prompts medical attention. Early recognition of this link in primary care can be vital, as the underlying problem may be serious. These three conditions together explain most cases encountered in general practice.

Beyond them lie a range of less frequent but important conditions, particularly if first-line tests are unrevealing. Diabetes insipidus is the classic disorder producing water diuresis. In central diabetes insipidus, the hypothalamus or pituitary fails to produce or release sufficient antidiuretic hormone. This may follow head trauma, neurosurgery, or the presence of a tumour. In nephrogenic diabetes insipidus, the kidneys do not respond to antidiuretic hormone, whether due to inherited defects or, more commonly, acquired problems such as lithium therapy, chronic kidney disease, prolonged hypercalcaemia, or hypokalaemia. In both cases, the hallmark is persistent thirst and the passage of large volumes of very dilute urine.

Primary polydipsia is another mechanism, where excessive water intake produces increased output. It may be behavioural, sometimes linked to psychiatric illness, though it is also seen in otherwise healthy individuals who habitually consume large volumes of water believing it beneficial. Distinguishing this from diabetes insipidus can be challenging, and often requires further assessment in hospital. Other contributors include caffeine and alcohol, which promote diuresis and can tip susceptible patients into symptomatic polyuria. Post-obstructive diuresis, occurring after relief of long-standing obstruction, can be dramatic and requires careful fluid replacement. Chronic kidney disease, particularly of tubulointerstitial type, impairs concentrating capacity and leads to polyuria and nocturia. Less frequently, endocrine disorders such as Addison's disease or thyrotoxicosis may feature polyuria, though rarely as the main symptom.

The clinician must first establish whether the complaint represents true polyuria. A simple 24-hour urine collection or output diary often answers this question, and a daily volume consistently above three litres confirms the diagnosis. History-taking should cover duration, fluid intake, thirst, nocturia, and associated symptoms. Medication history is crucial, including prescribed diuretics, SGLT2 inhibitors, lithium, and over-the-counter remedies. Enquiry into alcohol and caffeine use is also important. Symptoms such as weight loss, recurrent infections, constipation, abdominal pain, bone pain, headaches, or visual changes may point towards specific causes. Examination should focus on hydration status, blood pressure, and pulse, while also looking for signs of systemic disease such as goitre, pigmentation, lymphadenopathy, abdominal masses, or palpable bladder.

Initial investigations in primary care are usually sufficient. Urinalysis will detect glucose, ketones, protein, or blood, while the specific gravity provides a rough guide to concentrating ability. Blood tests should include glucose, HbA1c, urea, electrolytes, creatinine, and corrected calcium. Thyroid function or cortisol testing can be added if the history raises suspicion. If basic assessment does not reveal the cause, or if rare conditions such as diabetes insipidus are suspected, referral is appropriate. In such cases, more detailed investigations are arranged in specialist settings. For the GP, it is enough to recognise the possibility and refer; the specifics of hospital tests need not concern the generalist.

There are several pitfalls to avoid. The first is mistaking urinary frequency for polyuria, a common error easily prevented by a simple diary.

The second is overlooking medication, especially when patients have recently started diuretics or SGLT2 inhibitors. The third is neglecting to check calcium and electrolytes, since hypercalcaemia and hypokalaemia can both impair concentrating ability and cause polyuria. Post-obstructive diuresis also deserves special care. The temptation may be to restrict fluids, but the correct approach is to replace urine output cautiously and monitor electrolytes. Finally, in patients with marked thirst, hypernatraemia, and very dilute urine, diabetes insipidus should be suspected, and urgent referral made, as dehydration can become life-threatening.

Polyuria is therefore a symptom that requires a structured and logical approach. In primary care, most cases are explained by diabetes mellitus, medication use, and hypercalcaemia. These must always be the first considerations. Less common causes, such as diabetes insipidus, primary polydipsia, post-obstructive diuresis, chronic kidney disease, and endocrine disorders, occur far less frequently but should not be forgotten. The distinction between primary care and specialist settings lies in the relative frequency of underlying causes. For the general practitioner, dealing confidently with the common while remaining alert to the uncommon ensures safe, efficient, and cost-effective care. By progressing logically from the likely to the rare, the clinician avoids unnecessary investigation while providing patients with clear answers and appropriate treatment.

Topic 6

Pruritus

Pruritus, or itching, is a common complaint in general practice and may arise from a wide range of causes. It can be localized to a particular area or generalized, and it may indicate a benign dermatological condition or serve as the earliest manifestation of systemic illness. The task for the clinician is to distinguish between the common, usually harmless causes and the more serious underlying conditions.

Chronicscratchingoftenleadstodistinctiveskinchanges.Prurigopresents as areas of depigmented scarring surrounded by hyperpigmentation, usually resulting from repeated scratching. Lichenification, caused by persistent rubbing, produces thickened and elevated patches of skin with a characteristic violet-brown colour. These chronically irritated areas are often referred to as lichen simplex or neurodermatitis. Localized pruritus may occur in specific sites, such as pruritus ani or pruritus vulvae, which are both frequent problems in primary care.

Generalized pruritus, particularly in the absence of a rash, should always prompt consideration of systemic disease. Obstructive jaundice is an important example and may arise from gallstones, carcinoma of the pancreas, primary sclerosing cholangitis, or primary biliary cholangitis. Cholestatic jaundice of late pregnancy and the rare pregnancy-related dermatosis known as herpes gestationis may also cause severe itching. Chronic renal failure is another well-recognised cause, often associated with Uraemia and secondary hyperparathyroidism. Endocrine disorders, including diabetes mellitus, hyperthyroidism, and hypothyroidism, can all contribute.

Malignant conditions such as Hodgkin lymphoma, pancreatic carcinoma, and cutaneous T-cell lymphoma including mycosis fungoides are sometimes heralded by itching before other symptoms appear. Haematological conditions such as leukaemia, polycythemia vera, and iron deficiency anaemia are also relevant. In addition, autoimmune connective tissue disorders such as scleroderma and dermatomyositis, malabsorption syndromes, and vasculitic disease may present with pruritus. Parasitic infestations, especially scabies and pediculosis, are well-known causes.

Localized itching is often the first presentation in primary care and may be due to scabies, pediculosis, eczema, urticaria, or fungal infections such as tinea or candidiasis. Pruritus ani may be caused by psoriasis, lichen planus, candidiasis, threadworm infestation, or contact dermatitis, while pruritus vulvae may result from candida infection, inflammatory dermatoses, or contact reactions.

From a practical perspective, the most common causes encountered in general practice are eczema, especially the atopic type in children, urticaria, scabies, and superficial fungal infections including candidiasis. In women, pregnancy-related dermatoses are another important consideration. Among systemic causes, obstructive jaundice, chronic renal failure, and haematological disorders such as polycythemia vera are the most significant. Malignancy must always be kept in mind in cases of persistent unexplained pruritus, particularly in older patients.

Diagnosis begins with a thorough history, covering duration, distribution, severity, associated skin changes, systemic symptoms such as weight loss, fever, or jaundice, and potential triggers such as food, medication, and environmental exposures. Family or personal history of allergy, systemic disease, or skin disorders may also be important. Physical examination requires careful inspection of the skin for primary lesions such as eczema, psoriasis, urticaria, scabies, or fungal infection. Secondary features of chronic scratching, such as excoriations and lichenification, should be noted. Systemic examination may reveal jaundice, lymphadenopathy, hepatosplenomegaly, or signs of thyroid disease.

Investigations should be guided by the clinical picture. In cases of generalized pruritus without rash, a basic screen including full blood count, renal and liver function, thyroid profile, blood glucose, iron studies, and inflammatory markers is appropriate. Depending on the presentation, additional tests may include autoimmune screening, chest X-ray, ultrasound, or skin scrapings to exclude infestation.

The principle of 'common is common' provides the most practical strategy. The majority of pruritus seen in primary care is due to common dermatological conditions such as eczema, urticaria, scabies, or superficial fungal infection, and these should always be considered first. When no primary skin disease is evident, the focus should move to systemic causes. The most frequent are liver disease, renal failure, and haematological disorders such as iron deficiency and polycythemia vera. Only when these are excluded should rarer causes, including malignancy, autoimmune disorders, and psychogenic or neurological conditions, be pursued.

Pruritus is therefore both a common and a complex presentation. For most patients it represents a benign condition, but in some it is the first clue to serious underlying illness. A careful structured approach, beginning with recognition of the common causes and proceeding step by step, ensures efficient, safe, and resource-conscious care

Topic 7

Palpitation

Palpitation, in clinical medicine, means being unusually aware of one's heartbeat. It is often described as pounding, thumping, fluttering, or racing in the chest. Some patients say it feels as if the heart skips or stops for a moment, while others feel strong, sudden blows inside the chest. These experiences differ from person to person, but they all mean the same thing – the patient has become aware of something that normally happens unnoticed. From a doctor's point of view, this is important because the heart beats about one hundred thousand times each day without attracting attention. When its pattern or force changes, the person becomes aware of it.

From the patient's side, the description is often less precise but equally important. Many describe a sense of worry, nervousness, or fear. Some feel frightened not because of pain or breathlessness, but because the feeling itself is strange and unsettling. Others mention heaviness in the chest, a sense of suffocation, or a need to sit up to breathe easily. Women going through menopause often link palpitations with hot flushes and night sweats, which disturb sleep and increase anxiety. Younger people may blame stress, emotions, or diet, and fear that this means heart disease. The doctor must understand these different perspectives so as not to dismiss the complaint or misunderstand the patient.

The approach to palpitation should always start with recognising the common causes before thinking about rarer ones. The list of possibilities is long, but practical diagnosis depends on focusing on what is most likely. Only when the everyday causes are excluded should rarer ones be considered, to avoid wasting time and missing the obvious.

Common causes include fever, anxiety, and simple sinus tachycardia. Fever is a classic cause because it naturally raises the pulse. A person with pneumonia, urinary infection, or even a mild viral illness may notice palpitations. Anxiety is perhaps the most frequent non-cardiac cause. Panic attacks can appear suddenly, with pounding heartbeats, sweating, trembling, and fear of death. The mechanism is overactive nerves and stress hormones, not a heart problem. This is common in general practice, where patients often seek reassurance.

The menopausal state deserves special mention. Palpitations can appear with hormonal changes and cause distress, even without heart disease. They often happen along with hot flushes, mood swings, or poor sleep. Although harmless, they may lead to repeated visits, and a careful explanation is often more useful than many tests.

When the common causes have been ruled out, more complex heart rhythm problems must be considered. These include supraventricular tachycardia, atrial fibrillation, and ectopic beats. Atrial fibrillation, especially when it comes and goes, can cause sudden, irregular palpitations which alarm patients. Ectopic beats, whether from the atria or ventricles, are felt as single thumps or short bursts of disturbance in an otherwise normal rhythm. They are usually harmless but can be frightening, so detection on examination or ECG is important to rule out serious rhythm problems.

Premature beats are in fact a very common reason for isolated palpitations. They may occur in healthy people, triggered by stress, caffeine, or alcohol. The patient often describes a 'missed beat' followed by a strong thump as the rhythm resets. Here the doctor's reassurance, supported by appropriate but not excessive investigation, is essential.

For junior doctors and GPs, attention should focus on the common causes because they explain most cases. Fever, anxiety, heart failure, and systemic illness come first. Palpitations may signal worsening in a patient with existing heart disease or may point to thyrotoxicosis, where excess thyroid hormone speeds the heartbeat and causes tremor, weight loss, and nervousness. Severe inflammatory conditions, such as arthritis, can provoke palpitations, and occasionally neurological disorders like Parkinson's disease affect the body's automatic control, though these are rare in general practice.

The doctor must decide when to manage in primary care and when to refer to hospital. Supraventricular tachycardia and atrial fibrillation, for example, can be recognised in the surgery but need referral for full treatment. The GP's duty is to identify the problem, stabilise if needed, and refer appropriately. Trying to manage complex arrhythmias entirely in primary care is neither safe nor realistic.

Most cases, however, can be handled through good history, examination, and simple tests. The history should ask about onset, duration, frequency, triggers, and associated symptoms such as chest pain, dizziness, or breathlessness. Family and drug history may reveal clues such as stimulant use or thyroid disease. Examination should check pulse rate and rhythm, blood pressure, and any signs of general illness.

Basic investigations like ECG, thyroid function, and blood count often clarify the cause. Most palpitations can then be traced to common and usually harmless origins. Yet some patients continue to have symptoms without clear cause. In these cases, further tests may be needed. Ambulatory ECG (Holter) monitoring, echocardiography, or exercise tests can help, especially when the irregularity is not seen during the visit. Such cases belong in secondary care where cardiology expertise and facilities are available.

It is worth repeating that the right strategy always starts with the common and moves to the uncommon. This saves time, avoids unnecessary worry, and ensures sensible use of resources. To jump straight to rare causes risks confusion and alarm; to ignore serious conditions like arrhythmia or thyrotoxicosis risks harm. The skill lies in balancing these priorities through experience and sensitivity.

Palpitation should never be dismissed as trivial. Although often harmless, it can sometimes point to serious disease. At the same time, it should not be over-investigated without reason, which wastes effort and makes patients anxious.

The wise clinician keeps a balanced view - attentive to the complaint, methodical in assessment, careful in interpretation, and ready to refer when needed.

The message is clear: start with the common, confirm your findings, and investigate with purpose. This approach is cost-effective, time-saving, and clinically safe.

Topic 8

Headache

Headache is one of the most common reasons for a patient to visit a doctor. In most cases, there is no serious underlying cause, and the problem can be resolved through a careful history, thoughtful examination, and honest reassurance. For many patients this is enough to ease anxiety and rebuild confidence.

In everyday practice, examination findings are often normal, and diagnosis depends largely on the story the patient tells. However, physical examination should never be skipped. It is important not only to exclude serious disease but also to show the patient that their concern is taken seriously.

Headache can be classified in many ways, but in practical work it is best to focus on the most common patterns first. Tension-type headache and psychogenic headache are by far the most frequent. Patients often describe a tight, pressure-like band around the head, more uncomfortable than sharp. These headaches tend to come and go with stress, tiredness, or long periods of concentration. They usually improve with rest, relaxation, and hydration. Exploring the patient's emotional and social life can be revealing, as anxiety and stress are common triggers. Examination is usually normal, and reassurance with explanation often provides great relief.

Migraine is another major cause and can be more disabling. The pain is often throbbing and one-sided, though it can affect both sides. Attacks last from several hours to a few days and are usually accompanied by nausea, vomiting, or sensitivity to light and sound. Some patients experience an aura – flashing lights, zigzag lines, or temporary blind spots – while others may feel tingling, numbness, or brief weakness. Migraine can seriously affect work and family life, and it must be managed with both acute treatment and prevention, as well as attention to sleep, hydration, and trigger control.

Less common but important are vascular causes. High blood pressure can cause headaches, particularly when severe or new, but not every headache in a person with hypertension is caused by this. Temporal arteritis must always be considered in older adults who develop a new headache with scalp tenderness, jaw pain, or visual symptoms. This condition can cause blindness if untreated and needs urgent diagnosis and steroid therapy.

Raised intracranial pressure is another red flag. Brain tumours, metastases, abscesses, or chronic subdural haematomas can all cause progressive headache, often worse in the morning or on coughing or bending. There may be vomiting, blurred vision, or neurological signs such as weakness or speech change. A past history of cancer, especially breast, bowel, or lung, must raise suspicion of metastasis. These patients need urgent evaluation and referral.

Head injury is another familiar cause. Most post-traumatic headaches settle quickly, but in some people they persist as part of post-concussion syndrome, with poor concentration, irritability, and fatigue lasting for weeks or months. Supportive management with explanation and pacing is essential in these cases.

Headaches can also come from ENT or eye conditions. Sinusitis may cause facial pain, nasal blockage, and tenderness over the sinuses. Acute glaucoma causes severe eye pain, blurred vision, haloes around lights, nausea, and vomiting, and needs immediate referral to prevent loss of sight.

Another helpful way to classify headaches is by duration and tempo. Acute headaches appear over hours or days. A thunderclap headache that reaches maximum intensity within seconds is a red flag for subarachnoid haemorrhage and needs emergency investigation. Meningitis and encephalitis present with fever, neck stiffness, vomiting, and sensitivity to light. These require urgent hospital care. Cerebral venous thrombosis, though rare, should be considered in young patients with risk factors such as pregnancy or clotting disorders. Subacute headaches develop over two to eight weeks and may indicate increased pressure from a tumour, abscess, or subdural haematoma. Symptoms usually get worse with time and may include nausea, vomiting, or morning headache. Examination should include fundoscopy and neurological checks for papilloedema or weakness. Tuberculous meningitis can also present this way and must be considered in at-risk patients. Chronic headaches, lasting more than three months, are usually due to tension-type mechanisms or chronic migraine. Overuse of painkillers can make them worse. Management must address stress, sleep, mood, and lifestyle, as well as medication. Patients who rely too much on analgesics benefit from gradual reduction, while those with frequent migraines may need preventive drugs.

Diagnosis relies mainly on history. Key points include onset, duration, frequency, severity, triggers, and associated features such as vision changes, weakness, or fever. Ask about past illnesses, family history, and medication use. Examination should focus on blood pressure, optic discs, and a brief neurological check. A normal examination is reassuring in most primary headaches.

Investigations should be guided by suspicion. Blood tests such as full blood count, ESR, and CRP help detect infection or inflammation. A chest X-ray may help when tuberculosis or cancer is suspected. Brain imaging with CT or MRI is reserved for red-flag cases - those with sudden severe onset, new neurological deficit, papilloedema, seizures, or a major change in pattern. Avoiding unnecessary scans prevents anxiety and the problem of incidental findings, while still ensuring safety.

In practice, the best approach is to start with the common and move to the uncommon. Most headaches will be tension-type or migraine, and these should be managed first. When features or examination suggest something unusual, widen the scope to consider systemic, vascular, or intracranial causes. Older patients, those with systemic symptoms, immune problems, or a history of cancer always need careful assessment.

Referral should follow a clear pattern. Uncertainty after assessment, failure of treatment, or suspicion of serious causes such as temporal arteritis, subarachnoid haemorrhage, meningitis, raised pressure, or venous thrombosis must prompt early specialist referral. The aim in primary care is not to confirm every diagnosis but to recognise when help is needed quickly and safely.

Headache is common but demands clear thinking. By starting with the likely causes, staying alert to danger signs, and investigating only when necessary, doctors can offer reassurance, avoid missing serious illness, and use resources wisely. Patients feel listened to, tests have purpose, and care remains efficient. Headache may seem simple, but it remains one of the best tests of sound clinical judgment.

The message is clear: start with the common, remain alert for the serious, and investigate with purpose. This approach is cost-effective, time-saving, and clinically safe.

Topic 9

PUO

Pyrexia of unknown origin, or PUO, is defined as fever exceeding 38.3°C on multiple occasions, persisting for more than three weeks, and remaining undiagnosed despite a thorough history and careful clinical examination. It is not a disease in itself but rather a clinical syndrome with a wide range of potential underlying causes. The concept is important because it reminds clinicians that fever is a manifestation of many conditions, some trivial but others serious, and that premature labelling of a patient as having PUO risks delay in reaching the correct diagnosis.

The first lesson in approaching PUO is that failure to conduct a meticulous history and physical examination often results in wasted time and resources. When patients are labelled too early as PUO, it may trigger a cascade of costly, unfocused investigations which prolong uncertainty and cause unnecessary anxiety.

In contrast, a detailed and systematic history, combined with a comprehensive examination, remains the most effective strategy to direct further investigation. At every stage the clinician must balance thoroughness with economy, aiming to be both cost-conscious and time-efficient.

The role of the general practitioner in PUO is limited, since most patients eventually require hospital assessment. Nevertheless, awareness of the concept and familiarity with the major causes is valuable in primary care. The GP may be the first to identify important clinical clues, to raise suspicion of serious disease, or to refer patients for more advanced investigation. In today's world of global travel and migration, clinicians must also remain alert to tropical and geographically specific diseases which may otherwise be overlooked.

The causes of PUO are extensive, but infectious disease remains the most common category. Tuberculosis is the classic diagnosis, often presenting insidiously with prolonged low-grade fever, night sweats, cough, weight loss, or a history of exposure. Intra-abdominal abscesses or soft-tissue collections may produce persistent fever with localised pain or tenderness. Dental infections may be underestimated as a source of fever. Infective endocarditis is another key cause, producing fever, malaise, and sometimes embolic phenomena. Viral infections, including cytomegalovirus and HIV, may be implicated, while fungal infections such as histoplasmosis or aspergillosis should be considered in immunocompromised individuals.

Parasitic causes include malaria, toxoplasmosis, and visceral leishmaniasis, all of which are significant in travellers returning from endemic regions.

The second major group of causes is inflammatory and autoimmune disease. Systemic lupus erythematosus, rheumatoid arthritis, and various forms of vasculitis may all manifest initially as prolonged fever. Temporal arteritis in older patients can be particularly significant, as delay in diagnosis risks permanent blindness. Sarcoidosis, Crohn's disease, and other granulomatous conditions may also present in this way.

Neoplastic disease represents the third important group. Haematological malignancies such as lymphoma and leukaemia are well recognised, often accompanied by weight loss and night sweats. Solid tumours such as renal cell carcinoma and hepatocellular carcinoma may also present with unexplained fever. Metastatic disease can similarly cause persistent pyrexia even before the primary tumour is diagnosed.

A fourth group comprises miscellaneous causes. Familial periodic fever syndromes, such as familial Mediterranean fever, should be remembered in patients from certain ethnic backgrounds. Drug-induced hypersensitivity reactions may mimic PUO, with non-steroidal anti-inflammatory drugs and anti-epileptics among the common culprits. Factitious fever, in which patients deliberately manipulate temperature recordings, is rare but important to consider when the story is inconsistent or unusual.

Clues from the history are often decisive. In abscesses, pain and localised tenderness may dominate. Endocarditis may be suggested by fever in a patient with a murmur, prosthetic valve, or history of intravenous drug use, especially when embolic signs are present. HIV infection should be suspected in those with persistent fever, lymphadenopathy, recurrent infections, or unexplained weight loss, particularly with relevant risk factors. Malaria is typically associated with cyclical fever, jaundice, and recent travel to endemic regions without prophylaxis.

Autoimmune disease may be suggested by rashes, joint pains, photosensitivity, or systemic malaise. Temporal arteritis may manifest with headache, scalp tenderness, or visual disturbance. Sarcoidosis may be suspected when cough, erythema nodosum, and bilateral hilar lymphadenopathy are found together. Malignancy should be considered when there is painless lymphadenopathy, hepatosplenomegaly, haematuria, or weight loss. Drug reactions may be suspected when fever follows the introduction of a new medication.

Examination is equally critical. Careful general observation can yield valuable clues: weight loss, skin rashes, clubbing, or visible lymphadenopathy may all provide diagnostic direction. Examination of the head and neck should include inspection of the eyes, mouth, and palate, looking for jaundice, uveitis, or oral ulcers. Lymph nodes should be palpated thoroughly.

Cardiovascular assessment may reveal murmurs or peripheral signs of endocarditis. Respiratory examination may identify crackles, dullness, or effusions pointing to infection or malignancy. Abdominal examination may detect organomegaly, masses, or localised tenderness suggesting abscess or tumour. Musculoskeletal examination may reveal synovitis or tenderness suggestive of autoimmune disease, or bony pain hinting at osteomyelitis or metastasis. Neurological assessment may uncover confusion or cranial nerve abnormalities, which could indicate meningitis, encephalitis, or intracranial mass lesions. Extremities should be examined for oedema or rashes.

Investigations should always be guided by clinical suspicion rather than pursued indiscriminately. Initial laboratory work typically includes a full blood count, looking for anaemia, leukocytosis, or cytopenias. Inflammatory markers such as ESR and CRP are valuable in gauging systemic activity. Urinalysis may reveal proteinuria or haematuria, suggesting renal disease or glomerulonephritis. Serological tests, such as antinuclear factor or rheumatoid factor, can support autoimmune diagnoses. Cultures of blood, urine, and other relevant fluids are mandatory.

Imaging may begin with chest radiography, which can reveal tuberculosis, sarcoidosis, or malignancy. Ultrasound or CT of the abdomen and pelvis may uncover abscesses, masses, or lymphadenopathy. More advanced tests, including MRI or PET scanning, may be required in unresolved cases. Biopsy of lymph nodes, bone marrow, or other suspicious tissue can ultimately provide the definitive diagnosis.

Despite the wide range of possibilities, a relatively small group of conditions account for most cases. Tuberculosis, HIV infection, deep-seated bacterial abscesses, infective endocarditis, autoimmune conditions such as rheumatoid arthritis and SLE, and malignancies such as renal cell carcinoma and lymphoma represent the bulk of diagnoses. For this reason, clinicians are advised to focus first on these common causes before embarking on an exhaustive search for rare conditions.

For the general practitioner or junior doctor, the most practical strategy is to begin with a thorough history and careful examination, focusing on exposure to tuberculosis, travel to endemic areas, sexual history, drug exposure, family background, and systemic symptoms. Physical examination should be unhurried and comprehensive, covering lymph nodes, heart sounds, chest, abdomen, musculoskeletal system, and nervous system.

Only when this foundation is secure should investigations proceed, beginning with simple blood tests, urine analysis, and chest radiography, and expanding only as the clinical picture dictates.

By narrowing the focus initially to the most likely causes, the clinician saves time and resources, avoids overwhelming the patient with unnecessary tests, and maximises the chance of making a timely and accurate diagnosis. PUO reminds us that fever without explanation should never be dismissed, but that it must be approached with discipline. The physician's greatest tools remain careful listening, thorough examination, and thoughtful interpretation of clues. Investigations are important, but they should always serve the clinical reasoning process rather than replace it.

Above all, PUO challenges the clinician's patience and persistence, reminding us that careful clinical reasoning remains the cornerstone of medicine.

Topic 10

Polyarthritis

Polyarthritis, meaning inflammation of several joints, is a common reason for patients to seek medical help. The main symptoms are pain, swelling, and stiffness, but the underlying causes are varied. The first task for the clinician is to decide whether the problem is confined to the joints or part of a wider systemic illness.

At first presentation, the diagnosis can be difficult, especially if the features are vague. However, a careful history, physical examination, and selected investigations usually provide the answer. The way in which the joints are affected - their pattern of involvement - is often the key.

A good history is more than a list of symptoms. It should identify timing, distribution, and associations. Rheumatoid arthritis usually develops slowly, with intermittent swelling and aching that may last for months or years. In contrast, systemic lupus erythematosus or some vasculitides may appear much more quickly, within weeks. Always ask about the exact onset of symptoms - it can be the single most useful clue.

The behaviour of the joints during the day also helps. Inflammatory arthritis is marked by long morning stiffness that improves with activity. Mechanical pain, as seen in osteoarthritis, becomes worse with use and eases with rest. Do not forget to ask about the duration of morning stiffness, as this often separates inflammatory from mechanical disease.

The pattern of joint involvement is another important clue. Rheumatoid arthritis typically affects the small joints of the hands and wrists in a symmetrical way, sparing the very end joints of the fingers. Osteoarthritis often affects weight-bearing joints and produces bony swellings such as

Heberden's and Bouchard's nodes. Gout usually begins in the big toe, but in advanced disease can involve several joints. Psoriatic arthritis may be asymmetrical and is often linked with psoriasis, nail pitting, or onycholysis. Always examine the skin and nails - missing psoriasis can mean missing the diagnosis.

Polyarthritis rarely occurs in isolation. Systemic features often point towards the cause. A butterfly rash across the cheeks suggests lupus. Painful red nodules on the shins may indicate sarcoidosis, inflammatory bowel disease, or a post-streptococcal reaction. Eye inflammation, such as uveitis, is strongly linked with spondyloarthropathies like ankylosing spondylitis or reactive arthritis. Chronic diarrhoea with arthritis suggests inflammatory bowel disease. Do not forget to look beyond the joints - systemic features are often the deciding factor.

Despite the wide range of possibilities, most cases in everyday practice fall into four groups: osteoarthritis, rheumatoid arthritis, gout, and psoriatic arthritis. Always consider these first before moving to rarer causes.

Osteoarthritis is common in older patients and typically involves the hips, knees, and hands. Pain worsens with use, improves with rest, and systemic features are absent. X-rays usually show narrowing of joint spaces and osteophyte formation.

Rheumatoid arthritis has a different character. It causes symmetrical joint inflammation, especially in the hands, and is often associated with fatigue and anaemia. Blood tests such as rheumatoid factor and anti-CCP antibodies support the diagnosis, while X-rays may show erosions and bone loss near the joints.

Gout is due to excess uric acid. It often begins with sudden painful swelling in the big toe but may become polyarticular in chronic disease. Raised uric acid levels and, more definitively, urate crystals in joint fluid confirm the diagnosis.

Psoriatic arthritis is closely linked with psoriasis and nail changes. It often has an asymmetrical pattern and may present with dactylitis, where entire fingers or toes are swollen.

If these typical patterns are not present, other causes must be considered.

Viral arthritis, such as that caused by parvovirus B19, hepatitis B, or rubella, can mimic autoimmune disease but usually improves on its own. For example, a young person presenting with joint pains after a viral illness may recover fully without specific treatment.

Bacterial infection usually affects one joint, but in immunocompromised patients it may involve several. This must always be suspected when joints are hot, swollen, and the patient is unwell. Never delay aspiration and antibiotics when infection is possible.

Lyme disease, caused by Borrelia burgdorferi, may lead to migrating or recurrent arthritis months after a tick bite. A history of a circular rash or travel to an endemic area is an important clue.

Sarcoidosis may present with arthritis alongside lung disease and skin lesions.

Juvenile idiopathic arthritis is an important diagnosis in children and young adults.

Connective tissue diseases and vasculitis, such as lupus or polyarteritis nodosa, can also present with polyarthritis as part of a wider systemic illness.

Investigations confirm and refine the diagnosis. Inflammatory markers such as ESR and CRP show disease activity. Rheumatoid factor and anti-CCP support rheumatoid arthritis. ANA and anti-dsDNA help identify lupus. Serum urate is measured when gout is suspected. Joint aspiration can confirm crystal arthritis or exclude infection with Gram stain and culture. Imaging adds further evidence: X-rays show joint space loss, osteophytes, or erosions; ultrasound detects synovitis and effusions; MRI is sensitive for early inflammatory and soft tissue change.

The clinical approach is stepwise. History defines onset, distribution, and systemic associations. Examination identifies inflamed joints and extra-articular signs. Investigations are then used to confirm the likely diagnosis, beginning with the common causes. Only when these are excluded should attention move to rarer conditions, supported by more specialised tests.

In practice, most cases can be explained by osteoarthritis, rheumatoid arthritis, gout, or psoriatic arthritis. Concentrating on these first saves both time and cost. Less common causes should be considered only when these are excluded.

The key is pattern recognition. Symmetrical small-joint disease suggests rheumatoid arthritis. Distal joint involvement with psoriasis points to psoriatic arthritis. Mechanical pain with bony enlargement is typical of osteoarthritis. Sudden acute attacks with urate crystals confirm gout. Systemic features such as rashes, diarrhoea, or eye inflammation guide the clinician toward lupus, inflammatory bowel disease, or a spondyloarthropathy.

By following this structured and cost-effective approach - history, examination, targeted investigations, and attention to systemic features - the complex field of polyarthritis becomes manageable. Most patients fit into familiar patterns, while rarer diagnoses reveal themselves with time, careful observation, and selective testing.

Topic 11

Visual Failure

Impairment of vision is a common presentation in clinical practice. In many patients it is due to simple refractive errors, which are easily corrected. However, other causes – some linked to systemic disease – require a broader and more structured approach. A careful history, detailed examination, and appropriate investigation are essential to identify the cause and prevent further loss.

In the UK, the main causes of blindness are cataracts, age-related macular degeneration, glaucoma, and diabetic retinopathy. These eye diseases usually progress slowly and are often detected through screening or routine checks. The key first step in assessment is to establish whether the visual loss is gradual or sudden, as this distinction immediately narrows the likely diagnosis.

The most frequent causes of visual failure are senile cataracts, age-related macular degeneration (AMD), chronic glaucoma, and diabetic retinopathy. These generally develop gradually, though each has its own clinical pattern.

Cataracts remain the leading cause of blindness worldwide. Patients describe gradual, painless blurring of vision, often likened to looking through mist or frosted glass. Glare, especially at night, is common. Examination reveals lens opacity, making the diagnosis straightforward. Cataract surgery is highly effective and provides excellent visual recovery. Always consider cataract first in older patients with gradual, painless visual decline.

Age-related macular degeneration (AMD) is another major cause in the elderly. It affects central vision, making reading and face recognition difficult. Patients may notice distortion of straight lines or a dark central patch (scotoma). Dry AMD progresses slowly with drusen and retinal atrophy, whereas wet AMD causes rapid loss through abnormal new vessel formation. Early recognition is vital, as anti-VEGF therapy for wet AMD can preserve sight. Always ask elderly patients about distortion or central blurring.

Chronic glaucoma is often called the 'silent thief of sight'. It causes progressive optic nerve damage with gradual loss of peripheral vision advancing towards the centre. Raised intraocular pressure is a major risk factor, but normal-tension glaucoma also occurs. Because early disease is often silent, many cases are detected only during routine optometry checks. Treatment may involve drops, laser, or surgery. Ask about family history, as risk increases among relatives.

Diabetic retinopathy is the leading cause of blindness in working-age adults. It develops from the microvascular complications of diabetes, causing retinal damage and abnormal vessel growth. Symptoms include blurred vision, floaters, or sudden loss from bleeding into the eye or retinal detachment. Regular screening and timely treatment – with laser or anti-VEGF injections – are essential. Always check for diabetes in any patient with unexplained visual problems.

While most visual failure develops gradually, some conditions cause sudden loss and need urgent attention. These are less common, but carry a high risk of permanent blindness if missed.

Retinal artery occlusion presents with sudden, painless, unilateral blindness. The retina appears pale with a cherry-red macula. This is an ophthalmic emergency requiring immediate referral to try to restore blood flow and prevent permanent loss.

Retinal vein occlusion usually causes sudden blurring, rather than total blindness. The fundus shows dilated veins, haemorrhages, and cotton-wool spots. Management focuses on treating underlying vascular risk factors such as hypertension and diabetes.

Optic neuritis, often associated with multiple sclerosis, typically affects young adults. Vision becomes reduced, with pain on eye movement and loss of colour perception. Neurological assessment and MRI are required. In a young person with sudden loss of vision and pain, optic neuritis should always be suspected.

Retinal detachment presents with flashing lights, floaters, or the feeling of a curtain coming across the vision. This is a surgical emergency, as prompt repair can restore sight. Always ask about these warning symptoms.

Assessment begins with a careful history. Establish whether vision loss is unilateral or bilateral, sudden or gradual, and whether it is painful or painless. Gradual, bilateral decline points to cataracts, AMD, glaucoma, or diabetic retinopathy. Sudden, unilateral loss raises concern for vascular occlusion, optic neuritis, or retinal detachment.

Examination should include visual acuity, visual fields, pupillary reactions, and fundoscopy. Systemic signs are also important: check blood pressure, look for carotid bruits, or murmurs suggesting embolic disease. Tenderness over the temporal artery in an older patient should always raise suspicion of giant cell arteritis, which needs urgent corticosteroid treatment to prevent irreversible blindness.

Investigations are guided by the likely diagnosis. Check blood glucose and HbA1c for diabetes. Measure ESR and CRP when giant cell arteritis is suspected. Optical coherence tomography (OCT) is useful for macular disease, while MRI helps diagnose optic neuritis. Cost-effective practice means starting with the common causes and reserving complex or expensive tests for unusual cases.

Visual failure is a common but potentially devastating symptom. In practice, most cases arise from cataracts, AMD, glaucoma, or diabetic retinopathy. These should always be considered first, since early recognition and treatment can prevent blindness and save resources.

Less common but urgent causes such as retinal artery occlusion, retinal detachment, and optic neuritis must not be overlooked, even though they are rarer. Delay in diagnosis can mean permanent loss of sight.

By following a structured approach – history, examination, focusing first on the common causes, and reserving specialised tests for atypical cases – clinicians can practise efficiently, safely, and cost-effectively.

The message is clear: always consider the common causes first, recognise emergencies without delay, and investigate with purpose. This approach is cost-effective, time-saving, and clinically safe.

Topic 12

Dyspnoea

Managing dyspnoea requires not only medical knowledge but also clinical intuition developed through experience. A systematic, patient-centred approach allows the clinician to narrow an overwhelming range of possibilities into a clear and manageable differential.

A useful starting point is classification by onset. Acute, subacute, and chronic presentations each have hallmark causes which guide diagnosis. Acute dyspnoea always demands urgent consideration of life-threatening conditions such as pulmonary embolism, pneumothorax, or left ventricular failure. Subacute breathlessness often arises from systemic illness such as anaemia or malignancy. Chronic dyspnoea, on the other hand, is usually linked to long-term disorders such as chronic obstructive pulmonary disease (COPD), interstitial lung disease, or obesity. Always begin by asking the patient how long they have been short of breath, as this simple question immediately frames the likely causes.

History remains the foundation of assessment. Associated symptoms such as fever, chest pain, haemoptysis, or wheeze may point directly toward infection, embolism, or airway disease. Past medical history, comorbidities, and previous episodes provide valuable context. Listening attentively not only refines the diagnosis but also reassures the patient and builds trust. Remember that careful questioning often reveals the diagnosis before any investigation is performed.

Examination remains indispensable, even in an era dominated by technology. Hyperresonance on percussion may suggest pneumothorax, bilateral crepitations indicate pulmonary oedema, and unilateral leg swelling can raise suspicion of deep vein thrombosis. A systematic physical examination can often narrow the diagnosis rapidly and cheaply. Never overlook these basic signs – they may provide the very clues that imaging later confirms.

Investigations should then be chosen judiciously. A chest X-ray is often the first and most informative test, identifying pneumonia, pneumothorax, or pleural effusion immediately. D-dimer testing can exclude pulmonary embolism in low-risk patients, but excessive use in those with little pre-test probability only generates unnecessary cost and follow-up scans. CT pulmonary angiography has transformed diagnosis but should be reserved for cases with strong indications. Blood tests such as full blood count and arterial blood gases add further pieces to the puzzle. The balance lies in using investigations to confirm what history and examination have already suggested, rather than as a scatter-gun search.

Cost-effectiveness must always remain central to good practice. Classifying dyspnoea by duration, listening carefully to the history, examining thoroughly, and reserving advanced investigations for cases where they are truly needed not only saves resources but also protects the patient from unnecessary procedures. Thoughtful clinical reasoning remains the most cost-effective investigation available.

Another essential aspect is continuous learning. Medicine evolves, and so must the clinician. New biomarkers, high-resolution imaging, and evolving management strategies continue to refine the assessment and treatment of dyspnoea. Yet the core principles remain unchanged: take a careful history, perform a structured examination, and apply investigations wisely. Experience provides the backbone, but adaptability ensures safe and modern practice.

Dyspnoea is one of the most common symptoms encountered in both primary and secondary care. It may be benign, but it can also signal life-threatening disease. A structured approach transforms this challenge into a manageable clinical pathway. Always begin by defining the time course, then consider the common causes first – COPD, heart failure, infection, anaemia, or obesity. From there, extend the scope to less common but critical conditions, such as pulmonary embolism or pneumothorax.

Above all, remember that dyspnoea is a symptom, not a diagnosis. The goal is not only to relieve the patient's breathlessness but to uncover and address its underlying cause. By combining clinical experience with a systematic method, the physician provides care that is efficient, cost-effective, and safe. This structured way of thinking saves valuable time and ensures that the most common and urgent causes are recognised first before rarer possibilities are explored.

The message is clear: define the onset, identify the common causes first, and investigate with purpose. This approach is cost-effective, time-saving, and clinically safe.

Topic 13

Children: Bruising and Bleeding

Bruising and bleeding are common presentations in children and often cause anxiety for both parents and clinicians. The key challenge lies in distinguishing harmless causes from those that require urgent attention. A structured approach not only ensures diagnostic accuracy but also avoids unnecessary testing, reduces anxiety, and keeps clinical practice efficient and cost-effective.

An important first step is understanding the basic terms. Purpura are small haemorrhages in the skin, appearing as flat, purple spots that do not blanch with pressure. They reflect bleeding beneath the skin due to capillary fragility.

Ecchymosis (plural, ecchymoses) is the medical term for bruising, larger purpuric patches with well-defined borders, also non-blanching and usually due to capillary fragility. Bruises or contusions represent bleeding into the subcutaneous tissue and are often caused by trauma. Unlike purpura, they do not necessarily reflect vessel fragility and may arise from either normal knocks and falls or from bleeding disorders such as haemophilia.

Understanding these distinctions is essential, as they form the foundation for sound clinical reasoning and effective communication with families.

The next step is to consider the possible causes. Broadly, bruising and bleeding in children may result from medical conditions, trauma, medications, or – more rarely – from nutritional or genetic factors.

Bleeding disorders such as haemophilia or von Willebrand disease often present early in life and may appear as recurrent or disproportionate bleeding after minor injury. Thrombocytopenia is another common cause, whether triggered by viral infection, immune processes, or bone-marrow infiltration.

Leukaemia and other marrow-failure states can present subtly with unexplained bruising alongside systemic features such as fever, pallor, fatigue, lymphadenopathy, or hepatosplenomegaly.

Trauma remains the most frequent explanation, but distinguishing accidental from non-accidental injury is critical. Accidental bruises usually occur on exposed or bony areas such as the shins, elbows, or forehead, particularly in active children. Non-accidental injury must always be suspected when bruises are found in unusual sites - for example, on the back, abdomen, or face - or when they form a recognisable pattern.

The child's age and developmental stage also provide context. A non-mobile infant with multiple bruises raises immediate concern. Clinicians must stay alert to these possibilities, and careful observation of the history, the explanation given, and parental behaviour may reveal inconsistencies that warrant safeguarding action.

Medications are another factor. Drugs which interfere with clotting - such as aspirin, non-steroidal anti-inflammatory drugs, or anticoagulants - may predispose to bruising even after minimal trauma. Genetic conditions can also present in subtle ways: while some are well recognised, others may cause bleeding without a clear syndromic picture. Nutritional deficiencies, particularly of vitamins C and K, are uncommon but should not be overlooked.

The approach to a child with bruising and bleeding must begin with a thorough history. Always ask directly about trauma, clarifying whether it was accidental or possibly inflicted. Enquire about the onset, duration, and evolution of bruises, and whether they appear frequently or without obvious cause. Ask about systemic symptoms such as fever, fatigue, or pallor; family history of bleeding; recent infections; and medications.

A careful examination follows, noting the distribution, size, and age of bruises; the presence of purpura or petechiae; and any associated findings such as lymphadenopathy, hepatosplenomegaly, or pallor.

Investigations should then be guided by the most likely diagnosis. A complete blood count with differential is usually the starting point, providing information about anaemia, platelet count, or white-cell abnormalities. Reticulocyte count and peripheral smear give further insight into marrow function and cell morphology. Coagulation studies – including prothrombin time, activated partial thromboplastin time, and fibrinogen – assess clotting pathways.

Liver-function tests may reveal underlying hepatic impairment. When abnormalities persist or suggest more serious pathology, further investigations such as imaging for organomegaly or bone-marrow examination may be required.

Throughout this process, the guiding principle must be efficiency and focus. As the old saying reminds us, 'common things are common, rare things are rare.' Always begin by considering the frequent explanations – trauma, thrombocytopenia, and common bleeding disorders – before pursuing more unusual conditions. This structured thinking not only avoids unnecessary testing but also builds confidence for both clinician and family.

Bruising and bleeding in children can appear alarming, but a methodical approach transforms a potentially overwhelming problem into a manageable diagnostic pathway. The clinician should always start with the common causes, considering trauma, simple bleeding disorders, and infection-related thrombocytopenia before entertaining rarer conditions.

If these are excluded and the picture remains unclear, then – and only then – is it reasonable to pursue unusual diagnoses such as malignancy, nutritional deficiencies, or rare genetic disorders.

This is the essential guidance for navigating complex presentations: begin with what is most probable, move step by step, and let the pattern of history, examination, and initial investigations direct the course. Always remember that this strategy is not only clinically sound but also cost-effective and profoundly time-saving. In paediatrics especially, where both patient safety and family anxiety are paramount, avoiding unnecessary investigations is as important as identifying the rare but serious conditions.

In summary, efficiency, structure, and prioritisation of the common before the rare form the backbone of good paediatric practice. Applied with diligence and compassion, this structured, common-before-rare approach ensures safe, timely, and resource-conscious care for every child.

Topic 14

Lower Limb Weakness

Lower limb weakness is a common but often challenging presentation in everyday practice. The key to approaching it successfully is to follow a clear, structured pathway that begins with the most frequent and treatable causes before expanding to less common conditions. This exercise is not simply about listing possibilities: it is about teaching the clinician how to navigate quickly and safely to the correct diagnosis in a manner that is cost-effective and time-saving.

In most patients, the explanation lies within a familiar group of conditions. Osteoarthritis, particularly in older adults, restricts movement through pain and stiffness, resulting in reduced mobility and secondary muscle weakness. Trauma, whether from fractures, ligament injuries, or soft tissue damage, produces obvious loss of function that is usually apparent from history and examination.

Stroke remains a major cause, presenting with sudden unilateral weakness and often other neurological signs, and always requiring urgent recognition. Diabetes contributes significantly through peripheral neuropathy, which leads to bilateral weakness accompanied by sensory disturbance and imbalance.

By considering these four conditions first – osteoarthritis, trauma, stroke, and diabetic neuropathy – the clinician addresses the majority of cases in a logical and efficient way.

When these common explanations are excluded, attention turns to broader possibilities. Neurological disorders such as spinal cord compression, multiple sclerosis, or Guillain-Barré syndrome may present with progressive or acute weakness. Here the tempo of onset and the presence of sensory or sphincter involvement provide vital clues.

Muscular diseases form another important category. Polymyositis typically presents with proximal weakness and raised muscle enzymes, while inherited muscular dystrophies present earlier in life but should remain in the differential.

Vascular conditions can also affect limb power. Peripheral arterial disease produces claudication and reduced endurance, while venous obstruction leads more to swelling and heaviness than to true loss of strength.

Systemic and metabolic disorders must also be remembered. Endocrine disease such as hypothyroidism, vitamin B12 and vitamin D deficiencies, and electrolyte disturbances including hypokalaemia can all manifest as weakness. These causes are often reversible if recognised early.

Finally, in some cases no structural pathology is present and the weakness may be functional or psychological, reminding clinicians to approach every patient with balance and sensitivity.

A thorough history is the starting point. The time course, pattern of progression, associated symptoms, and relevant medical or lifestyle factors provide direction. A history of alcohol misuse suggests nutritional neuropathy, while known malignancy may indicate spinal cord involvement.

Examination then builds on this foundation. Spasticity and exaggerated reflexes point to central causes; wasting and fasciculations indicate peripheral or muscular disease; diminished pulses or limb swelling highlight vascular compromise.

Investigations are guided by clinical judgement, rather than performed indiscriminately.

Simple blood tests may reveal anaemia, thyroid dysfunction, or electrolyte imbalance. Imaging, whether plain X-ray, ultrasound, or MRI, is used selectively when structural or vascular disease is suspected. Electrophysiological studies such as nerve conduction tests are reserved for situations where a neuromuscular disorder is genuinely suspected.

By tailoring investigations in this way, care remains both accurate and efficient, avoiding unnecessary costs or delays.

The essence of managing lower limb weakness lies in balancing thoroughness with practicality. Common and treatable conditions must always be considered first, as they account for the bulk of cases. Clinicians must also remain alert to less frequent but serious disorders where prompt intervention can be life-saving.

This structured approach ensures that patients receive timely and appropriate care, while investigations remain focused, safe, and cost-effective.

In summary, lower limb weakness is best understood as a clinical exercise in disciplined reasoning. By starting with the most common causes and expanding logically outward, the clinician achieves an approach that is efficient, accurate, and protective of patient safety.

The message is clear: always start with the common causes, expand logically, and investigate with purpose. This approach is cost-effective, time-saving, and clinically safe.

Topic 15

Congestive Heart Failure (CHF)

Congestive heart failure is a common condition and one of the most rewarding to diagnose and treat effectively. The syndrome itself is often recognised with ease, but the real challenge is to identify the cause. Correctly identifying the underlying problem not only directs treatment but also prevents unnecessary investigations and saves valuable time and resources.

The majority of patients present with one of four common causes. These should always be considered first.

Ischaemic heart disease is the leading cause worldwide. A history of angina, myocardial infarction, or coronary intervention usually provides a clear link. The failing ventricle, weakened by infarction or chronic ischaemia, can no longer maintain output.

Hypertension is the next most frequent cause. Long-standing, uncontrolled blood pressure places a constant burden on the myocardium. Over time the left ventricle becomes thickened, then stiff, and eventually weak, leading to failure.

Valvular disease must also be remembered. Severe aortic stenosis, aortic regurgitation, or mitral regurgitation can all result in progressive strain on the heart. In settings where rheumatic heart disease is prevalent, valve lesions are particularly important.

Arrhythmias, especially atrial fibrillation, complete the group of common causes. They disrupt coordinated filling, reduce cardiac efficiency, and often trigger decompensation.

When these four causes - coronary artery disease, hypertension, valvular disease, and atrial fibrillation - are not evident, the clinician must widen the differential. Other cardiac problems such as dilated or hypertrophic cardiomyopathy, congenital heart defects, and pericardial disease may be responsible. In each case, the history, age of the patient, and associated features provide important clues.

Non-cardiac causes are less frequent but still significant. Chronic obstructive pulmonary disease (COPD) and pulmonary hypertension place a strain on the right ventricle. Severe anaemia can produce high-output failure. Thyrotoxicosis accelerates metabolism and increases cardiac demand. Diabetes, alcohol misuse, certain drugs, and viral myocarditis are additional contributors, particularly in patients without the usual cardiac risk factors.

Symptoms usually guide the clinician quickly. Breathlessness is the hallmark, appearing at first with exertion but later even at rest. Orthopnoea - the inability to lie flat without becoming breathless - is particularly suggestive. Many patients describe waking at night gasping for air, a classic feature known as paroxysmal nocturnal dyspnoea. Fatigue, reduced exercise tolerance, and ankle swelling are common, while advanced cases may show ascites, weight gain, or muscle wasting.

On examination, typical findings strengthen the suspicion. Raised jugular venous pressure, basal lung crepitations, and peripheral oedema are all important. A displaced apex beat indicates cardiac enlargement. Murmurs suggest valve disease, while an irregularly irregular pulse points to atrial fibrillation. Each finding is helpful, though none is diagnostic in isolation.

Investigations then confirm and refine the diagnosis. Natriuretic peptides (BNP or NT-proBNP) are sensitive markers of cardiac stress and help prioritise further testing. Echocardiography is the key test, providing direct assessment of ejection fraction, valve abnormalities, and chamber size. Chest X-ray may reveal cardiomegaly or pulmonary congestion. The ECG can show arrhythmias, ischaemia, or previous infarction. Blood tests identify systemic factors such as thyroid disease, anaemia, electrolyte disturbance, or renal impairment.

Advanced tests - such as coronary imaging, stress testing, or cardiac catheterisation - are reserved for selected cases where ischaemic disease is suspected or the mechanism of failure remains uncertain despite initial evaluation.

A structured approach ensures efficiency. Begin with the four most common causes - coronary artery disease, hypertension, valvular disease, and atrial fibrillation. If none of these is apparent, look outward to cardiomyopathies, pericardial disease, or congenital problems, and only then to non-cardiac and rarer causes. This order of thought saves time, prevents unnecessary tests, and directs resources where they matter most.

Accurate diagnosis is essential because treatment depends on cause. Coronary disease may require revascularisation. Hypertension needs strict control. Valvular disease may demand intervention. Arrhythmias require rhythm or rate control and anticoagulation. Identifying and correcting precipitants - such as thyrotoxicosis, anaemia, infection, excess salt, or alcohol - may reverse decompensation entirely. Without this focus, management risks being incomplete, limited to symptomatic relief while the disease continues unchecked.

In summary, congestive heart failure is best approached as a teaching exercise in structured clinical reasoning. Start with the four common causes, then move step by step through the less frequent cardiac and non-cardiac explanations. Combine history, examination, and selective investigations to confirm the diagnosis and define the mechanism. The message is clear: begin with the common, expand logically, and investigate with purpose. This approach is cost-effective, time-saving, and clinically safe.

Topic 16

Changes in Bowel Habits

Changes in bowel habits are a frequent reason for consultation in both primary and secondary care. They may result from something as simple as a dietary change or may signal serious disease such as colorectal cancer. The challenge for the clinician is to distinguish the common and benign from the dangerous and urgent. This requires a structured approach guided by careful history-taking, thoughtful examination, and selective investigation.

In most cases, the explanation lies within a straightforward group of causes. Dietary change, low fibre intake, poor hydration, or the use of constipating or laxative medications often account for the symptoms. Functional bowel disorders, such as irritable bowel syndrome or functional constipation, are also extremely common. Infective causes explain many acute cases, particularly after travel, recent illness, or ingestion of contaminated food. Most of these conditions can be managed with reassurance, dietary advice, and simple treatment, without the need for extensive testing.

When these common explanations are not evident, the clinician must look further. Inflammatory bowel disease, such as Crohn's disease or ulcerative colitis, presents with diarrhoea, weight loss, fatigue, abdominal pain, and sometimes fever. Neoplastic disease is of particular concern: colorectal cancer may first present as persistent alteration in bowel habits, often with rectal bleeding, anaemia, or unexplained weight loss. In these patients, urgent investigation is essential.

Systemic and metabolic conditions can also affect bowel function. Hyperthyroidism often produces diarrhoea, while hypothyroidism slows gut motility and leads to constipation. Diabetes may disturb bowel rhythm through autonomic neuropathy. Neurological diseases such as Parkinson's disease or spinal cord disorders can alter bowel activity. Vascular causes, including ischaemic colitis, usually occur in older patients and present with sudden abdominal pain and bloody diarrhoea.

Psychological and emotional factors frequently aggravate functional symptoms. Stress and anxiety are well-known triggers of irritable bowel disturbance. Recognising this connection is important, since unnecessary investigation of purely functional symptoms wastes resources and increases patient anxiety.

The key teaching point is to always distinguish routine from urgent cases. Red flag features must be actively sought: unexplained weight loss, rectal bleeding, persistent abdominal pain, iron-deficiency anaemia, or a family history of colorectal cancer or inflammatory bowel disease. The presence of any of these should move the case immediately into the urgent category. Ignoring red flags or dismissing them as 'functional' is a mistake to be avoided.

History and examination remain the foundation of diagnosis. The duration and progression of symptoms, associated systemic features, drug use, travel history, and family history all guide suspicion. Examination may reveal anaemia, weight loss, abdominal tenderness, or a palpable mass. A rectal examination should never be omitted, as it may reveal tumours, fissures, or impacted stool.

Investigations must be chosen with care. Simple tests such as full blood count, inflammatory markers, and thyroid function are often sufficient to narrow the differential. Stool cultures may identify infection. Faecal calprotectin helps distinguish inflammatory bowel disease from functional disorders, and faecal occult blood testing may detect hidden bleeding. Coeliac serology should be included when gluten sensitivity is suspected.

Imaging and endoscopy are powerful, but must be used judiciously. An abdominal X-ray may show obstruction or faecal loading. CT or MRI is valuable when masses or inflammatory disease are suspected.

Colonoscopy remains the gold standard for diagnosing colorectal cancer, polyps, or inflammatory bowel disease, but it should be performed only when indicated, as it carries cost, risk, and patient burden.

The teaching message is clear: do not investigate every patient with minor or self-limiting symptoms. This wastes resources, exposes patients to unnecessary procedures, and delays attention to those who truly need urgent care. Instead, begin with the common causes, manage and reassure where appropriate, and reserve advanced investigations for patients with red flag features or persistent, unexplained change.

In summary, changes in bowel habits are best approached with disciplined, structured reasoning. Begin with the frequent causes - diet, medication, infection, and functional disorders. Always be vigilant for red flags which demand urgent referral for colorectal cancer or inflammatory bowel disease. Use history, examination, and selective investigations to guide decisions, avoiding indiscriminate testing.

This approach is efficient, clinically safe, and cost-effective, ensuring that patients receive timely and appropriate care while valuable resources are used wisely.

Topic 17

Steatorrhea and Malabsorption

Steatorrhea refers to the passage of pale, bulky, foul-smelling stools which are often difficult to flush. It occurs when fat is poorly absorbed and passes into the stool in excess. Malabsorption is a broader condition, involving defective absorption of nutrients such as fats, proteins, carbohydrates, vitamins, and minerals. Steatorrhea is therefore best regarded as a visible sign of fat malabsorption, often drawing clinical attention to an underlying disorder.

Malabsorption arises when normal digestion or absorption is disrupted at one or more levels - within the intestinal lumen, at the mucosal surface, or during nutrient transport. The clinical task is to recognise this syndrome early, focus on the most frequent causes, and investigate in a structured way. Doing so ensures that patient care is accurate, safe, time-saving, and cost-effective.

In clinical practice, a small number of conditions account for most cases. Coeliac disease is one of the leading causes. It often presents with diarrhoea, bloating, weight loss, and iron deficiency. Chronic pancreatitis is another common culprit, usually associated with long-term alcohol misuse, but also with genetic or metabolic factors. Crohn's disease is an important differential, in which inflammation and scarring of the small intestine limit absorption.

Other frequent causes include bile acid deficiency, often following ileal resection or disease, and lactose intolerance, which typically causes diarrhoea, bloating, and discomfort after dairy products. Drug-induced malabsorption must also be remembered, with orlistat being the best-known example. These six conditions - coeliac disease, chronic pancreatitis, Crohn's disease, bile acid deficiency, lactose intolerance, and drug-related malabsorption - account for the majority of cases and should always be considered first.

Less common causes include pancreatic cancer, biliary obstruction from gallstones, primary biliary cholangitis, cystic fibrosis in children and young adults, and a variety of rare congenital or metabolic disorders. These should be investigated only after the common culprits have been excluded, or when the clinical picture is atypical.

The patient's history often provides the most valuable clues. Alcohol misuse suggests chronic pancreatitis. Jaundice, pruritus, or a history of gallstones raise suspicion of biliary obstruction. Chronic diarrhoea with blood or abdominal pain may indicate inflammatory bowel disease. Bloating and floating stools after dairy products point strongly toward lactose intolerance. Reviewing medications is essential, as drug-induced malabsorption is frequently overlooked.

Examination reveals the systemic consequences of malabsorption. Weight loss despite a normal appetite is a key diagnostic clue. In children, poor growth or failure to thrive may be the first sign. Protein deficiency leads to muscle wasting and oedema. Fat-soluble vitamin deficiency produces characteristic manifestations: night blindness from lack of vitamin A, bone pain or fractures from vitamin D deficiency, easy bruising from vitamin K deficiency, and neuropathy or ataxia from vitamin E deficiency. Recognising these signs directs both diagnosis and treatment.

Investigations should proceed step by step. Stool fat analysis is a simple starting point, whether by Sudan stain or a timed stool collection. Once malabsorption is confirmed, targeted tests help determine the cause. Coeliac serology is highly useful, while stool elastase is the investigation of choice for pancreatic insufficiency. Tests for bile acid loss may be required in selected patients.

Imaging plays a supportive role. Ultrasound or CT can identify chronic pancreatitis, biliary obstruction, or malignancy. MRCP and ERCP are reserved for cases where ductal disease is suspected. Endoscopy with duodenal biopsy remains essential for confirming coeliac disease and may also reveal other small bowel pathology.

The guiding principle is to follow a structured, stepwise pathway. Start with history and examination, then confirm malabsorption with simple stool tests. From there, move to targeted investigations based on the most likely cause. Only escalate to advanced imaging or invasive procedures when needed. Indiscriminate testing wastes resources, increases patient burden, and delays appropriate treatment.

Red flags must always be considered. Persistent, unexplained weight loss, severe or worsening diarrhoea, evidence of protein–calorie malnutrition, fat-soluble vitamin deficiency with systemic consequences, or unexplained anaemia should all prompt urgent and thorough evaluation. These features may indicate an underlying malignancy, advanced inflammatory bowel disease, or significant pancreatic or biliary pathology. Ignoring them risks missing serious and potentially treatable conditions.

Clinicians must also remember what not to do. Do not dismiss unexplained weight loss or micronutrient deficiency as irritable bowel syndrome. Do not overlook dietary or drug causes, as these are among the most common and easily treatable. And do not over-investigate mild, self-limiting symptoms when the history clearly points to a benign cause such as lactose intolerance.

In summary, steatorrhea and malabsorption are best approached through structured clinical reasoning. The clinician should first consider the common causes – coeliac disease, chronic pancreatitis, Crohn's disease, bile acid deficiency, lactose intolerance, and drug-induced malabsorption. Careful history and examination then guide selective investigations. This approach ensures timely, accurate, and cost-effective diagnosis, avoids unnecessary procedures, and prevents the long-term complications of untreated malabsorption.

The message is clear: think of the common causes first, work systematically, and use resources wisely.

Topic 18

Dizziness

Dizziness is a frequent complaint in clinical practice and yet one of the most imprecise terms used by patients. It can describe a range of sensations, including lightheadedness, unsteadiness, or the spinning sensation of vertigo. Because the word is vague, the first and most important step for the clinician is to clarify what the patient actually means when they say they feel dizzy.

For some, dizziness reflects a sense of movement within themselves, while for others it is a perception that their surroundings are moving. A true rotational sensation is better described as vertigo and usually indicates a disorder of the vestibular system. Non-vertiginous dizziness, on the other hand, may arise from cardiovascular, neurological, metabolic, or psychological causes. Sorting this out quickly and accurately is crucial to avoid unnecessary tests and to direct the patient toward thc correct pathway of care.

In day-to-day practice, most patients presenting with dizziness have one of a small number of common conditions. Benign paroxysmal positional vertigo (BPPV) is perhaps the most frequent. It produces brief episodes of vertigo triggered by changes in position, such as turning in bed or bending forward. Most patients respond well to simple repositioning manoeuvres, and the condition should not be over-investigated once the diagnosis is clear.

Ménière's disease and vestibular neuritis are also important causes. Ménière's disease presents with recurrent episodes of vertigo accompanied by hearing loss, tinnitus, and a sense of aural fullness. Vestibular neuritis typically follows a viral illness and produces severe vertigo that may last for days, but in many cases improves gradually with supportive care. Together, these disorders account for the majority of vertiginous presentations seen in practice.

Other causes, while less frequent, must still be kept in mind. Central nervous system disease, such as stroke, multiple sclerosis, or posterior fossa tumours, may present with dizziness, usually accompanied by other neurological deficits. Cardiovascular conditions are another important group. Arrhythmias, postural hypotension, or autonomic dysfunction reduce cerebral perfusion and lead to presyncopal dizziness. Psychological causes, including anxiety and panic disorder, are also common, especially when dizziness is accompanied by a feeling of detachment or fear. Recognising these patterns early prevents wasteful investigations and ensures timely intervention.

The clinical approach must always begin with a careful history. Patients should be encouraged to describe their symptoms in their own words. The clinician should determine whether the sensation is truly rotational or more like faintness or imbalance. The timing and duration of episodes are critical: seconds suggest BPPV, hours point towards Ménière's disease, and days suggest vestibular neuritis. Sudden and persistent dizziness with associated neurological features must immediately raise concern for a cerebrovascular event. Triggers such as position change, exertion, or emotional stress often provide valuable diagnostic clues.

Examination then confirms or refines the working diagnosis. Neurological assessment may reveal nystagmus, cranial nerve abnormalities, or incoordination. Simple bedside tests such as the Dix-Hallpike manoeuvre, head impulse test, and Romberg test are cost-effective tools that often make expensive investigations unnecessary. Cardiovascular examination is equally important, since orthostatic hypotension or an irregular pulse may provide the answer without delay.

Investigations should be chosen selectively and never ordered indiscriminately. Audiometry is useful when hearing loss accompanies vertigo. Neuroimaging, usually MRI, is reserved for patients with suspected central pathology such as stroke or tumour. Blood tests are guided by clinical suspicion, checking for anaemia, electrolyte disturbance, or thyroid disease. Electrocardiography should be performed if an arrhythmia is suspected. By tailoring tests to the clinical picture, clinicians avoid unnecessary cost, minimise delays, and preserve resources.

The teaching point is that most cases of dizziness can be diagnosed with a structured history, focused examination, and minimal investigation. The majority of patients will prove to have BPPV, Ménière's disease, vestibular neuritis, or cardiovascular-related dizziness. Recognising these conditions promptly is not only safe but also highly cost-effective, as it prevents unnecessary imaging and hospital referrals. Do not over-investigate or over-emphasise dizziness when the diagnosis is already clear.

Red flags, however, must never be ignored. Sudden dizziness with severe headache may signal a stroke or subarachnoid haemorrhage. Persistent vertigo accompanied by neurological deficits suggests central disease and demands urgent attention. Progressive hearing loss or unsteadiness may indicate tumours or degenerative disorders. The presence of these features should always prompt urgent referral and investigation.

In summary, dizziness is a broad and often confusing symptom, but most cases arise from a few common causes which can be identified with careful questioning and simple examination. By clarifying what the patient means, focusing on the common conditions first, and using investigations selectively, clinicians can provide safe, time-saving, and cost-effective care. At the same time, vigilance for red flags ensures that serious disease is never overlooked. This structured approach demonstrates the balance of efficiency and accuracy that lies at the heart of good clinical practice.

Topic 19

Facial Pain

Facial pain is a common but complex clinical presentation. It can arise from a wide spectrum of causes, ranging from benign everyday conditions to serious underlying disease. Because of this variety, clinicians must adopt a systematic approach. The focus should always begin with the common and likely causes, before considering the rarer possibilities. This strategy is both safe and cost-effective, ensuring that patients receive timely treatment while avoiding unnecessary investigations.

In daily practice, migraine is one of the leading causes of facial pain. It often produces throbbing or pulsating discomfort that may spread across the face. The pain is frequently accompanied by nausea, sensitivity to light, or overwhelming fatigue. These features, together with its recurrent pattern, usually make the diagnosis clear.

Dental infection or abscess is another major cause. Pain is typically sharp and localised, often worsening with chewing or pressure. Swelling and tenderness are common, and sometimes the source is obvious on oral examination. Prompt recognition is vital, as untreated dental infection can spread beyond the oral cavity.

Temporomandibular joint dysfunction (TMJ disorder) is also frequently encountered. It produces pain in the jaw, temple, or ear, often aggravated by talking, chewing, or yawning. Clicking, popping, or restricted jaw movement may be detected on examination, confirming the diagnosis without further tests.

Sinusitis is another frequent explanation, presenting with dull, pressure-like pain over the affected sinus. It is often accompanied by nasal congestion or discharge. In acute cases, fever may be present, while chronic sinusitis may produce more subtle and persistent symptoms.

Shingles and post-herpetic neuralgia are less common but highly characteristic. Severe burning or tingling pain, sometimes following the distribution of the trigeminal nerve, is a key feature. Pain may persist long after the rash has healed, and its neuropathic quality is usually unmistakable.

Once these common causes are addressed, attention turns to less frequent but important differentials. Trigeminal neuralgia is a classic example. It produces sudden, electric shock-like bursts of pain, usually confined to one side of the face and often triggered by light touch, chewing, or speaking. Though less common, it is highly characteristic and should not be confused with other disorders.

Cluster headache may also present with severe, one-sided facial pain around the eye, accompanied by tearing or nasal congestion. Musculoskeletal syndromes, such as myofascial pain, may refer discomfort from the neck or shoulders into the face. On rare occasions, pain may even be referred from distant sites such as the ear or heart, with angina sometimes manifesting as pain in the jaw.

The cornerstone of diagnosis remains a careful and structured history. The quality of the pain is often decisive: throbbing suggests migraine; sharp and localised pain with swelling points to a dental abscess; burning pain after a rash is typical of post-herpetic neuralgia; and pressure with congestion is seen in sinusitis.

Timing is equally important. Migraines are episodic, dental pain persists until treated, and trigeminal neuralgia is brief but recurrent. Identifying triggers adds further clarity. Chewing may worsen temporomandibular pain, stress may provoke migraine, and even light touch may precipitate trigeminal neuralgia. Associated symptoms such as fever, rash, or nasal discharge complete the clinical picture.

Examination should then confirm the suspicion raised by history. Swelling and tenderness are usually obvious in dental or sinus disease. Restricted jaw movement or clicking indicates to temporomandibular dysfunction. A rash or residual scarring along the trigeminal distribution confirms shingles. Neurological assessment may reveal sensory loss, hyperalgesia, or cranial nerve abnormalities, which help distinguish neuropathic causes.

Investigations must be used selectively. Most cases of facial pain can be diagnosed through history and examination alone. Simple blood tests may confirm systemic infection or inflammation. Imaging, such as MRI or CT, should be reserved for suspected structural disease, tumours, or vascular lesions. Electrophysiological studies may be appropriate only in complex cases of neuropathic pain. Avoiding indiscriminate testing reduces costs, prevents unnecessary anxiety, and streamlines care.

The main teaching message is that, despite its wide differential, facial pain most often arises from a limited group of common and recognisable conditions. By focusing on these first – migraine, dental infection, sinusitis, temporomandibular dysfunction, and shingles – the clinician can make a diagnosis quickly and accurately without extensive investigation. Rarer conditions such as trigeminal neuralgia or vascular disorders should only be pursued when history and examination support them.

Red flags must always be considered. Unexplained persistent facial pain, neurological deficits such as numbness or weakness, progressive swelling, weight loss, or systemic illness should prompt urgent and thorough evaluation. These features may signal malignancy, intracranial pathology, or advanced infection, and should never be dismissed.

In summary, facial pain is a diagnostic challenge but one that can be managed effectively with a structured and logical approach. Clinicians should begin with the most common causes, use history and examination as their primary tools, and reserve investigations for selected cases. This approach not only saves time and resources but also ensures patient safety. Above all, the goal is precision without excess: accurate diagnosis, cost-effective investigation, and timely treatment.

Topic 20

Urine Examination

Urine examination is one of the simplest and most useful diagnostic tools in medicine. It provides rapid, non-invasive information about kidney function, metabolic health, and systemic disease. Because it is quick, inexpensive, and highly informative, it continues to play a central role in clinical practice, especially in primary care, where it can save time, reduce unnecessary referrals, and offer safe, cost-effective care.

The physical appearance of urine is often the first clue. Normal urine is pale yellow to amber, depending on hydration. Cloudy urine may suggest pus, crystals, or bacterial infection. Red or pink urine often indicates blood, which may come from stones, trauma, infection, or malignancy. Brown or tea-coloured urine points to bile pigments or myoglobin, raising suspicion of liver or muscle disease. Even odour can be diagnostic: a strong ammonia smell suggests infection, while a fruity odour is typical of uncontrolled diabetes.

The dipstick test is the most practical and widely used part of urinalysis. It is inexpensive, quick, and provides immediate results. Protein on the dipstick may indicate kidney disease, though transient traces are sometimes seen after fever or exertion. Glucose is normally absent; its presence suggests diabetes or renal tubular dysfunction. Ketones indicate fasting, starvation, or diabetic ketoacidosis, which is a medical emergency.

Blood detected by dipstick is important, though not always straightforward: it may represent true haematuria, haemoglobin, myoglobin, or contamination during collection. Nitrites and leukocyte esterase are particularly valuable. When positive in a patient with dysuria, urgency, or frequency, they strongly suggest a urinary tract infection (UTI).

Microscopic examination adds further precision. The presence of red blood cells confirms haematuria, while increased white blood cells support infection or inflammation. Casts are highly informative. Red cell casts point towards glomerulonephritis, white cell casts are typical of pyelonephritis, and granular or waxy casts suggest chronic kidney disease. Crystals also carry diagnostic weight. Calcium oxalate indicates stone disease, uric acid crystals are seen in gout or hyperuricaemia, and cystine crystals suggest rare metabolic disorders.

In everyday practice, urine testing is most often used to detect infection. A dipstick positive for leukocytes or nitrites, alongside compatible symptoms, can establish the diagnosis of a urinary tract infection within minutes. It is also a valuable tool in monitoring chronic disease. In diabetes, the detection of glycosuria or ketonuria may indicate poor control or dangerous metabolic decompensation. In kidney disease, persistent proteinuria provides an early warning of deterioration. Pregnancy testing is another common application, as the presence of hCG in urine is an inexpensive and reliable diagnostic marker.

The method of sample collection matters. A midstream clean-catch sample reduces contamination and improves accuracy. In selected situations, such as assessing daily protein excretion or creatinine clearance, a 24-hour collection is needed. However, this is less convenient for patients and prone to error if the collection is incomplete.

Interpretation of results should always be careful and based on the patient's overall situation. A single abnormal finding is not always significant. Transient proteinuria may follow exertion or fever. Isolated haematuria may occur after vigorous exercise. The key point is persistence. Repeated proteinuria should be confirmed with quantitative testing, while recurrent haematuria requires imaging or cytology to exclude stones or malignancy. Abnormal pH values should raise the possibility of systemic acid-base disturbance.

The strength of urine examination lies in its efficiency. With one simple test, a clinician can detect infection, monitor diabetes, identify kidney disease, or uncover systemic illness. Because the dipstick provides immediate results at low cost, it remains one of the most time-saving investigations in medicine. Used wisely, it guides further testing without encouraging unnecessary or wasteful investigations.

Red Flags

Certain findings in urine examination must never be ignored. Persistent haematuria may indicate malignancy. Significant proteinuria often points to underlying renal disease. The presence of ketones in a patient with diabetes is a sign of potential ketoacidosis, which is a medical emergency. These situations demand urgent investigation and timely referral.

In summary, urine examination is a cornerstone of clinical practice. Observation of colour and clarity, dipstick testing for blood, protein, glucose, ketones, leukocytes, and nitrites, and microscopic assessment for cells, casts, and crystals together offer a broad yet practical evaluation of health. Above all, the dipstick is the most powerful tool: it allows rapid, cost-effective detection of the common problems - urinary infection, diabetes, and kidney disease. Interpreted correctly, urinalysis saves time, avoids unnecessary investigations, and continues to provide a reliable path to early diagnosis.

Topic 21

Chest Pain

Chest pain is one of the most frequent presentations in both emergency and general practice. Its importance lies not only in how common it is but also in how easily a life-threatening condition can be overlooked if the assessment is not systematic. The clinician's aim should be to concentrate on the common and critical causes first, using history, examination, and a small number of targeted tests. This ensures safe, time-saving, and cost-effective care.

The evaluation begins with a clear and focused history. The character of the pain, its site, duration, radiation, and relation to exertion or meals are vital clues. Associated features such as breathlessness, sweating, palpitations, cough, fever, or haemoptysis may point towards a particular system. Past medical history - including cardiovascular disease, reflux, recent surgery, or risk factors such as smoking and immobility - must always be sought. A careful history often narrows the possibilities without the need for extensive investigation.

Examination is equally important. Vital signs - pulse, blood pressure, temperature, and oxygen saturation - immediately show how unwell the patient is. Cardiovascular assessment may reveal murmurs, gallops, or raised jugular venous pressure. Chest examination can detect crepitations, pleural rubs, or absent breath sounds. Reproducible pain on palpation of the chest wall strongly suggests a musculoskeletal cause. These observations, though basic, remain the most time-saving and cost-effective tools.

The most important diagnosis to prioritise is ischaemic heart disease. Angina and myocardial infarction typically cause central, heavy, or crushing pain, sometimes radiating to the jaw or arm, and often accompanied by sweating, nausea, or collapse. Because delay can be fatal, an ECG and troponin should be obtained early. These simple and inexpensive tests are critical in confirming or excluding the diagnosis.

Respiratory disease is the next key category. Pneumonia often produces pleuritic pain with fever, cough, and sputum. A chest X-ray is a straightforward, inexpensive test that confirms the diagnosis. Pulmonary embolism, though less common, must be suspected when pain and breathlessness occur suddenly, particularly in patients with recent immobility, surgery, or malignancy. Clinical scoring systems and a D-dimer test guide the need for imaging, avoiding unnecessary scans in low-risk patients. Pneumothorax presents with sudden, sharp pain and breathlessness; again, a chest X-ray provides rapid diagnosis.

Gastro-oesophageal reflux disease (GERD) and oesophageal spasm are frequent mimics of cardiac chest pain. A burning retrosternal discomfort, symptoms related to meals, or relief with antacids are typical features. Recognising this pattern prevents needless investigations and inappropriate admissions.

Musculoskeletal chest pain, such as costochondritis or muscle strain, is also common. It presents with sharp, localised pain that is reproducible on palpation. In the absence of systemic or cardiac signs, this diagnosis can be made confidently at the bedside, avoiding further tests.

Other causes are less frequent, but should remain in mind. Aortic dissection produces sudden, severe, tearing pain radiating to the back, sometimes with pulse or blood pressure differences. Pericarditis causes sharp pain relieved by sitting forward, while pericardial rupture may present with shock. Oesophageal rupture, usually after forceful vomiting, is rare but catastrophic. Haemoptysis with chest pain suggests pulmonary embolism or malignancy. Herpes zoster may present as burning pain before the rash appears. These conditions are uncommon, but awareness of their features prevents missed diagnoses.

Investigations should always be guided by clinical suspicion. The ECG, cardiac enzymes, and chest X-ray form the foundation of assessment. Blood tests such as D-dimer are useful when carefully selected. Advanced investigations - CT, MRI, or endoscopy - should be reserved for cases where first-line assessment raises specific concerns. This strategy ensures safety while avoiding wasteful use of resources.

Red Flags

Red flags must be recognised immediately. Sudden severe chest pain, collapse, radiation to the jaw, arm, or back, haemodynamic instability, or associated haemoptysis demand urgent action. These are the features that signal life-threatening disease and must never be overlooked.

In summary, chest pain requires a disciplined, structured approach. The majority of cases arise from ischaemic heart disease, reflux, pneumonia, pulmonary embolism, or musculoskeletal pain. These must always be prioritised, as they account for most presentations. Less common but serious conditions should be remembered selectively, without overwhelming the clinician with unlikely diagnoses. By starting with history, focusing on examination, and using only the most informative investigations, clinicians can achieve safe, accurate, and cost-effective diagnosis, ensuring that patients with chest pain receive timely and appropriate care.

Topic 22

Leg Ulcers

Leg ulcers are common in clinical practice and create substantial morbidity through pain, infection, immobility, and social impact. A clear, economical approach prevents missed diagnoses and avoids waste. The aim is simple: start with the causes which explain most cases, use bedside clues, and reserve advanced tests for selected situations.

The great majority fall into three groups. Venous ulceration is the leading cause, driven by chronic venous insufficiency after valve failure or previous deep vein thrombosis. Arterial disease forms the next major group in people with peripheral vascular disease. Neuropathic ulcers, particularly in diabetes, make up the third. Mixed arterial-venous disease is also frequent. Rarer aetiologies - vasculitis, haematological disorders, malignancy, or chronic infections - should be considered only when the presentation is atypical or the usual causes do not fit.

History-taking sets the direction. Establish duration, rate of change, preceding trauma, and any prior ulcers. Ask about varicose veins, DVT, limb swelling, or long-standing oedema to support a venous origin. Claudication, rest pain, night pain relieved by hanging the leg over the bed, smoking, or known vascular disease suggest arterial insufficiency. In diabetes, elicit neuropathic symptoms, foot deformity, poor footwear, or prior ulceration. Pain characteristics help: venous ulcers cause mild discomfort eased by elevation; arterial ulcers are painful and worse on elevation; neuropathic ulcers may be painless.

Examination confirms the pattern. Venous ulcers are shallow, irregular, and typically lie in the gaiter area above the ankle. The surrounding skin may show hyperpigmentation, eczema, or lipodermatosclerosis, with ankle oedema and visible varicosities.

Arterial ulcers have sharply demarcated, 'punched-out' edges and may show dry necrosis or eschar. They occur on toes, heels, or pressure points. The limb is cool and pale, pulses are weak or absent, hair is sparse, and the skin is thin and shiny.

Neuropathic ulcers occur at pressure sites on insensate feet, especially the plantar surface and under metatarsal heads. Callus is common around the lesion. Test sensation with a monofilament or tuning fork; loss of protective sensation is a key clue.

In every patient, look for infection - erythema, warmth, swelling, malodour, or purulent discharge - and for systemic signs such as fever. Examine peripheral pulses, capillary refill, and for bruits. Note deformity, Charcot changes, and footwear. These bedside findings are the fastest, most informative, and most resource-conscious elements of the assessment.

Investigations should be chosen with care, because unnecessary testing wastes time and money. The ankle-brachial pressure index (ABPI) is the first-line study when arterial disease is a possibility. Values below 0.9 indicate arterial insufficiency; values above 1.3 suggest calcified, noncompressible vessels, common in diabetes, and call for toe pressures or waveform analysis.

Handheld Doppler assessment adds more detail of arterial signals and venous reflux. Duplex ultrasound maps venous incompetence when intervention is considered and assesses arterial flow when revascularisation might be needed. Use it when the result will change management.

Basic blood tests are targeted. Check glucose and HbA1c to detect or monitor diabetes. Full blood count and inflammatory markers help judge infection or systemic inflammation. Swab only when there is clinical infection; colonisation is frequent and indiscriminate swabbing drives unnecessary antibiotics.

Reserve advanced imaging for specific indications. CT or MR angiography is for patients with critical limb ischaemia who are candidates for revascularisation. Plain X-ray of the foot is useful if osteomyelitis is suspected. Biopsy any ulcer with atypical appearance, everted edges, exuberant granulation, or failure to heal despite appropriate care to exclude malignancy or vasculitis.

The diagnostic emphasis remains on the common patterns. In venous disease, the story is long-standing oedema, skin change at the ankle, and a shallow irregular ulcer in the gaiter area. In arterial disease, the picture is rest pain, a cold pulseless limb, and a sharply edged ulcer on toes or heels. In neuropathy, the hallmark is a plantar ulcer on an insensate foot with surrounding callus. Mixed disease shows features of more than one group; ABPI and Doppler help determine which element dominates and therefore which pathway to pursue.

Keep rare causes in mind, but briefly. Vasculitis may present with multiple painful ulcers and livedo; haematological disease can produce leg ulceration in sickle cell anaemia; squamous cell carcinoma may arise in long-standing wounds (Marjolin ulcer). Chronic atypical infection is uncommon in most settings but should be considered with relevant epidemiology. These diagnoses are exceptions; they should not distract from the common patterns unless the clinical picture demands it.

Red Flags

Rapidly enlarging ulcers, rest pain or acute limb ischaemia, black necrotic tissue with absent pulses, spreading cellulitis with systemic toxicity, suspected osteomyelitis, or features suggestive of malignant change demand prompt escalation and specialist referral. The presence of any of these should immediately shift the plan from routine evaluation to urgent management and definitive imaging or biopsy.

Throughout, remain disciplined about cost and time. ABPI and focused Doppler are inexpensive, quick, and answer the key question: arterial, venous, neuropathic, or mixed? Unselective use of cultures, broad imaging, or indiscriminate blood panels adds little and delays decisions. Let history and examination lead; use tests which confirm what you already suspect; escalate only when results will change management or a red flag is present.

In summary, leg ulcers are best approached by concentrating on venous, arterial, neuropathic, and mixed causes, because these explain most cases. Take a precise history, examine with intent, and use ABPI and targeted Doppler as your core investigations. Consider rarer aetiologies only when the presentation is atypical or the wound fails to behave as expected. By following this sequence - common first, tests which matter, red flags never missed - you deliver diagnosis that is accurate, timely, and resource-conscious.

Topic 23

Pleural Effusion

Pleural effusion is the abnormal accumulation of fluid within the pleural space. Normally, this space contains only a very thin film of fluid, enough to act as a lubricant so that the lungs expand and contract smoothly during breathing. The balance of production and absorption is tightly regulated by hydrostatic and oncotic pressures, as well as lymphatic drainage. When this balance is disturbed, fluid accumulates and produces clinical consequences.

Effusions are broadly divided into transudates and exudates. The distinction is based largely on protein content, with transudates containing less than 30 g/L of protein and exudates being protein-rich. This reflects their mechanism: transudates arise when systemic factors, such as raised hydrostatic pressure or reduced oncotic pressure, push fluid into the pleural cavity. Exudates occur when local disease processes increase vascular permeability or impair pleural clearance. In practice, Light's criteria are often applied to separate the two with greater accuracy, comparing pleural fluid with serum protein and lactate dehydrogenase.

Although management usually lies within hospital care, the role of the general practitioner (GP) is crucial. The GP suspects the condition, makes the initial diagnosis, arranges a chest X-ray, and refers appropriately. Early recognition matters because causes are diverse, and outcomes differ significantly.

The potential causes are many. Local pleural or pulmonary disease includes primary pleural malignancy, metastatic deposits, pneumonia, bronchiectasis, tuberculosis, fungal infection, and lung abscess. Trauma, thoracic surgery, oesophageal perforation, or a subphrenic abscess may also extend to the pleura. Systemic illness contributes as well, most often through heart failure, cirrhosis of the liver, nephrotic syndrome, or severe malnutrition. Autoimmune disease such as rheumatoid arthritis and systemic lupus erythematosus, or lymphatic obstruction due to thoracic malignancy, must also be considered.

Yet despite this wide range, in daily practice only a handful of conditions are seen most often. These are heart failure, liver cirrhosis, pulmonary embolism, lung cancer, and tuberculosis. Concentrating on this group saves time, prevents unnecessary investigations, and keeps the approach efficient and cost-effective.

History provides important clues. A patient recently discharged from hospital who becomes breathless may have a pulmonary embolism. A young woman on oral contraceptives with chest pain and dyspnoea raises the same suspicion. Weight loss, chronic cough, and smoking history suggest malignancy, while fever, night sweats, and prolonged cough point to tuberculosis. Past medical history also matters: cardiac disease or chronic liver disease often directs the diagnosis quickly towards transudative effusions. Even dietary and social history can be relevant, as malnutrition and alcoholism are established contributors.

Examination should be purposeful. The doctor should concentrate on signs which help guide the diagnosis. Clubbing, hepatosplenomegaly, lymphadenopathy, or joint disease may all be significant. Chest findings such as dullness to percussion and diminished breath sounds suggest the possible presence of pleural fluid but cannot confirm it. Only aspiration and analysis of pleural fluid can establish the diagnosis with certainty. Systemic features such as fever, cachexia, or long-standing illness may then help narrow the underlying cause.

Investigations follow the same reasoning. A chest X-ray is usually the first step and often shows a meniscus of fluid or a white-out of the lung base. Ultrasound of the chest can detect smaller collections and guide aspiration, while computed tomography (CT) provides further anatomical detail, especially where malignancy is suspected. Blood tests support the picture: a full blood count, inflammatory markers, liver function, renal profile, and serum proteins all add useful information. Pleural aspiration, performed in secondary care, provides the most specific evidence, with analysis of protein, LDH, glucose, pH, cytology, and microbiology. Cytology may confirm malignant cells, while culture or staining may reveal tuberculosis.

The principle is straightforward: do not become distracted by the many rare causes. Keep the common conditions in mind, direct the history and examination towards them, and arrange investigations which are relevant. Once this stage is complete, referral to secondary care ensures the patient receives definitive management.

Management itself is not the focus here, but in outline it depends on treating the underlying cause. Large effusions may be aspirated to relieve symptoms, yet the true priority is to diagnose and address the primary pathology, whether cardiac failure, malignancy, tuberculosis, or another condition. This responsibility rests with the hospital team, while the GP's task is early recognition, targeted investigation, and prompt referral.

In conclusion, pleural effusion can appear daunting because of the wide range of possible causes. With a structured and logical approach, however, it becomes manageable. The skill lies in filtering information, concentrating first on the most likely diagnoses, and building a clear diagnostic pathway. In doing so, the clinician saves time, reduces cost, and ensures patients receive the right care without delay. For junior doctors and general practitioners, the lesson is clear: always think of the common causes first, let them guide your reasoning, and keep your approach practical and purposeful.

Topic 24

Haemoptysis

Haemoptysis, the expectoration of blood from the respiratory tract, is a presentation that often causes fear and anxiety in patients and demands careful assessment by clinicians. It may occur in general practice, where it frequently prompts urgent consultation, or in hospital settings such as emergency departments and respiratory clinics. The sight of blood is naturally alarming, particularly for smokers or those with chronic lung disease, and it often brings patients directly to their doctor. Clinicians must balance reassurance with vigilance, as haemoptysis can represent anything from a benign, self-limiting problem to a serious and potentially fatal condition.

The very first step in approaching a patient with suspected haemoptysis is to establish whether the bleeding is truly originating from the lungs. This distinction is critical. Many patients assume that blood seen in their sputum must be coming from the chest, but in reality, bleeding may have arisen from several alternative sources. Blood from the lips, gums, or posterior nasal passages may be coughed up after trickling into the pharynx.

Epistaxis that tracks backwards into the throat can be swallowed and later vomited, giving a false impression of haemoptysis. Gastrointestinal bleeding may also be misinterpreted when blood is vomited. In children, swallowed foreign bodies occasionally cause airway trauma and subsequent blood-stained sputum. For this reason, careful questioning is essential to distinguish between true haemoptysis, pseudohaemoptysis, and haematemesis.

Once the source of bleeding is confirmed to be the lungs, a systematic history is the foundation of diagnosis. Important questions include the amount and frequency of blood, its duration, and whether it appears mixed with sputum or as pure blood. Associated symptoms must be elicited: cough, fever, chest pain, weight loss, or night sweats all provide diagnostic clues.

Smoking history is of prime importance, since chronic bronchitis, bronchiectasis, and carcinoma are all strongly associated with long-term tobacco exposure. Even patients who have recently stopped smoking may still be at risk of conditions which developed during their years of smoking.

Risk factors for pulmonary embolism should always be considered, particularly in young or middle-aged patients presenting with sudden onset haemoptysis. These include recent surgery, prolonged immobilisation, long-distance travel, pregnancy, and use of the oral contraceptive pill. A history of previous tuberculosis remains highly relevant, especially in individuals from endemic regions, as post-TB scarring and cavities can predispose to recurrent bleeding.

Cardiovascular conditions may also contribute. Pulmonary embolism is a significant and ongoing cause. Mitral stenosis, once a common culprit, has become rare in developed countries due to the availability of antibiotics and improved medical care, though it may still be encountered occasionally, especially in low-resource settings. Trauma – whether accidental or iatrogenic following procedures such as bronchoscopy – can also result in bleeding.

Clinical examination should follow a structured approach. General inspection may reveal finger clubbing, often associated with bronchiectasis, lung abscess, or carcinoma. Examination of the chest may uncover focal signs such as consolidation, collapse, or coarse crepitations. Wheeze or bronchial breathing may indicate underlying airway or parenchymal disease.

The cardiovascular examination is equally important. A mid-diastolic murmur may suggest mitral stenosis, while an irregularly irregular pulse points towards atrial fibrillation. Evidence of heart failure, such as ankle oedema or raised jugular venous pressure, should be sought. The lower limbs should also be inspected for swelling or tenderness that may indicate deep vein thrombosis, which in turn raises suspicion of pulmonary embolism.

Investigations must be guided by the clinical findings but usually start with chest radiography, which can demonstrate pneumonia, bronchiectasis, tuberculosis, or a pulmonary mass. Sputum examination for cytology and culture is helpful in identifying infective organisms or malignant cells. Blood tests, including full blood count, clotting profile, and inflammatory markers, provide additional information.

Where uncertainty remains, more advanced imaging is required. CT scan of the chest, CT pulmonary angiography, and ventilation-perfusion (V/Q) scans are now central to modern investigation. Bronchoscopy, although invasive, may be essential when bleeding is persistent, unexplained, or suspected to be due to a localised lesion such as carcinoma.

When considering the differential diagnosis, it is crucial to focus first on the common causes, since these account for the majority of cases in clinical practice. Respiratory causes dominate and include acute infections such as pneumonia and bronchitis, chronic suppurative conditions such as bronchiectasis, tuberculosis (old or active), and carcinoma of the lung.

Cardiovascular causes, particularly pulmonary embolism, must also be kept in mind. Haematological disorders which impair clotting, as well as chest trauma, are less common but should not be ignored. Rare causes, including vasculitis or autoimmune disorders such as Goodpasture's syndrome, may only be suspected once the more typical diagnoses have been excluded.

It is also useful to distinguish between minor and massive haemoptysis. Minor bleeding – for example, streaks of blood in sputum during a chest infection – is relatively common and often benign. However, even small amounts may signal a more sinister underlying condition in a smoker or in a patient with systemic symptoms.

Massive haemoptysis, usually defined as more than 200-600 mL of blood in 24 hours, is immediately life-threatening, due to the risk of airway obstruction and asphyxiation. In such cases, rapid hospital admission and specialist intervention are mandatory. This distinction underlines the importance of assessing not only the cause but also the severity of bleeding when first encountering the patient.

While management lies largely in secondary care, the role of the general practitioner or hospital doctor at first presentation is crucial. Identifying risk factors, recognising red flag features, and arranging timely referral can make the difference between life and death. In practice, the priority is always patient safety. It is far better to investigate thoroughly and refer early than to risk overlooking a serious underlying condition such as carcinoma, tuberculosis, or pulmonary embolism.

In conclusion, haemoptysis should never be dismissed. Although some causes are minor and self-limiting, others carry grave implications. A structured approach - confirming the source, taking a careful history, performing a thorough examination, and guiding investigations appropriately - is essential. Above all, attention must be directed first to the common and important conditions, ensuring patient safety remains the overriding priority.

Topic 25

Peripheral Oedema

Oedema is the abnormal accumulation of excess fluid within the interstitial spaces. It is a common clinical sign encountered in both hospital and general practice and should always prompt careful consideration of the underlying cause.

Patients often present with swelling of the ankles, feet, or sacral area, and in some cases with abdominal distension due to ascites. Because it can arise from many different mechanisms, a structured approach is required. History and examination usually provide the main clues, and when combined with targeted investigations, they guide diagnosis without unnecessary delay.

For clarity, oedema may be classified into four broad categories: generalised oedema due to salt and water retention, oedema caused by increased vascular permeability, oedema due to lymphatic obstruction, and oedema resulting from venous obstruction. Each group has typical causes and characteristic features, and distinguishing between them allows the clinician to focus on the most likely explanation.

The first mechanism - generalised oedema due to salt and water retention - is the most frequently encountered. Liver disease, heart failure, and renal pathology are the main culprits. In liver cirrhosis, the history may reveal alcohol intake, previous hepatitis B or C infection, or a background of hepatocellular carcinoma. Past surgery or travel to regions where schistosomiasis is endemic, particularly in the Middle East, may also be relevant. Such patients often present with ascites in addition to peripheral swelling.

Congestive heart failure is another major cause. The history should cover prior ischaemic events, valvular problems, and symptoms of breathlessness or reduced exercise tolerance. Oedema in this setting typically develops in dependent areas, such as the ankles or sacrum. Renal disease may also contribute, particularly in younger patients or those with connective tissue disorders such as systemic lupus erythematosus. A past history of proteinuria, steroid therapy, or renal biopsy may provide important clues, although in practice renal causes are less frequently seen than hepatic or cardiac ones. Malnutrition can also lead to hypoproteinaemia, reducing plasma oncotic pressure and resulting in widespread oedema.

The second mechanism is increased vascular permeability. Local infections such as cellulitis produce swelling that is warm, erythematous, and tender, helping to distinguish them from systemic causes. Allergic vasculitis, erythema nodosum, and polyarteritis nodosa may also present with swelling. Angioedema is another striking example, characterised by rapid swelling of the lips, eyelids, or larynx. Although often allergic, hereditary forms exist and may be accompanied by recurrent abdominal pain or, in severe cases, dangerous laryngeal obstruction.

The third mechanism is lymphatic obstruction. This may follow radiotherapy or surgery, particularly in association with breast carcinoma, and often progresses slowly due to lymphatic fibrosis. The resulting oedema is firm, non-pitting, and associated with thickened, brownish skin. This contrasts with the soft, pitting oedema of cardiac or hepatic origin. In tropical countries, filariasis remains a recognised cause, and travel history is therefore important.

The fourth mechanism is venous obstruction. Deep venous thrombosis (DVT) is common, and the history may reveal recent surgery, prolonged immobilisation, or use of the oral contraceptive pill. Venous obstruction is usually unilateral, although pelvic compression from an abdominal mass can lead to bilateral swelling.

Obstruction of the vena cava produces more widespread swelling. Superior vena cava obstruction results in oedema of the face and upper limbs, while inferior vena cava obstruction affects both legs. Diagnosis may be more difficult if the acute episode has already subsided, and careful questioning about earlier symptoms is often helpful.

On examination, the findings vary with the cause. In liver disease, stigmata such as spider naevi, palmar erythema, hepatomegaly, and flapping tremor may be present. In renal conditions, periorbital oedema may be particularly striking, while in cardiac failure the clinician may find raised jugular venous pressure, basal lung crepitations, and peripheral swelling. Lymphatic obstruction produces non-pitting oedema with skin thickening and fibrosis.

Drug history is crucial. Calcium channel blockers, frequently used for hypertension, are a well-known cause of ankle swelling. Withdrawal of the drug usually resolves the problem and prevents unnecessary investigations. Other agents, including certain anti-inflammatory drugs, can also contribute.

Investigations should be guided by the history and examination, rather than applied indiscriminately. Basic tests include renal function, liver function with albumin, urinalysis for proteinuria, and gamma-GT. Echocardiography is useful when cardiac disease is suspected, while Doppler ultrasound is essential in suspected venous thrombosis. More advanced investigations, such as immunological tests, biopsy, or imaging for malignancy, are reserved for cases where they are medically pertinent.

In everyday practice, the most common causes of oedema are congestive heart failure, liver cirrhosis, venous obstruction, and drug-induced swelling. Less frequent but still important causes include nephrotic syndrome and tropical infections such as filariasis.

It must be emphasised that a cost-effective approach is essential. This does not mean compromising standards of care, but rather beginning with the most likely and common causes. Careful history-taking and examination usually provide the main clues, and in many cases they point clearly to the diagnosis without the need for expensive or invasive investigations.

This approach reduces delays, saves healthcare resources, and avoids unnecessary patient anxiety.

Ultimately, the priority is always patient safety. Cost-effectiveness naturally follows when clinicians focus first on the common causes and use investigations selectively. This method ensures that care remains safe, clinically effective, and economically responsible.

Topic 26

Understanding Coma - Causes and Diagnostic Approach

A coma is a profound state of unconsciousness in which a patient cannot be awakened, fails to respond to painful stimuli, and shows no normal sleep-wake cycle. Consciousness depends on the proper function of two critical components of the brain: the reticular activating system, which regulates arousal, and the cerebral hemispheres, which generate higher thought processes. When either of these is damaged or disrupted, the patient may lapse into coma. This condition may arise from structural causes such as stroke, haemorrhage, or traumatic brain injury, or from non-structural causes such as metabolic disturbances, systemic infections, or intoxication.

The immediate priority in managing a comatose patient is stabilisation of vital functions. Airway patency, adequate breathing, and effective circulation must be secured before further steps can be taken. Oxygen is administered, and in many cases intubation is required to protect the airway and support ventilation. Circulatory status, blood pressure, and oxygen saturation are monitored closely, and abnormalities corrected without delay. Only once this urgent phase of care is complete can the focus shift towards identifying the underlying cause.

A careful neurological assessment follows stabilisation. The level of consciousness is often measured using the Glasgow Coma Scale, which provides a structured evaluation of eye opening, verbal response, and motor activity. Brainstem reflexes, including pupillary reactivity, corneal response, and oculocephalic movements, provide valuable information about brainstem integrity. Abnormal posturing or asymmetry in motor response may give further clues to the site and severity of injury. These bedside observations are crucial in distinguishing diffuse metabolic or toxic causes from structural lesions affecting specific regions of the brain.

Obtaining a detailed collateral history is another essential step. Because the patient is unable to provide information, accounts from relatives, friends, or emergency services become indispensable. Witness descriptions of collapse, seizure activity, head trauma, or substance ingestion may be critical. Past medical history of hypertension, diabetes, liver disease, or renal failure must be sought. Current medications, especially sedatives, opioids, or anticoagulants, may offer important clues. Exposure to toxins, recent infections, or alcohol use must also be explored.

The physical examination should be systematic, not limited to the neurological system. Signs of head trauma, meningism, fever, or systemic illness may guide the diagnostic process. A careful inspection for needle marks, jaundice, or signs of chronic disease may provide valuable direction.

Laboratory investigations are indispensable in the initial evaluation. Blood glucose is checked at once, since hypoglycaemia is a common and rapidly reversible cause. Serum electrolytes, renal function, and liver function tests may reveal metabolic derangements, while arterial blood gases help assess hypoxia, hypercapnia, or acidosis. If infection is suspected, blood cultures and, when safe, lumbar puncture with cerebrospinal fluid analysis are undertaken to identify pathogens. Toxicology screens are performed if overdose or poisoning is a possibility.

Imaging plays a central role when a structural lesion is suspected. A non-contrast CT scan of the brain is often the first choice because it rapidly identifies haemorrhage, infarction, or mass effect. MRI provides finer detail and is particularly valuable for diffuse axonal injury, posterior fossa pathology, or subtle cortical changes. Where vascular lesions are suspected, angiography can reveal aneurysms, malformations, or occlusions. Electroencephalography (EEG) may demonstrate seizure activity or diffuse encephalopathic patterns, particularly useful when non-convulsive status epilepticus is considered. In patients with suspected raised intracranial pressure, invasive monitoring may be employed to guide therapy.

Although coma has a wide differential diagnosis, several groups of causes are seen most frequently in daily practice. Structural injury to the brain is a leading cause. Traumatic brain injury, especially in younger adults, commonly results from road traffic accidents, falls, or assaults. The pathology may involve contusions, subdural or epidural haematomas, or diffuse axonal injury. A CT scan often confirms the diagnosis, and management may range from close monitoring to urgent neurosurgical intervention. Prognosis depends heavily on the severity of injury and the rapidity of treatment.

Cerebrovascular accidents are another major structural cause. Large ischaemic strokes can lead to extensive cortical or brainstem damage, while haemorrhagic strokes produce coma through mass effect and raised intracranial pressure. Both types require urgent neuroimaging for confirmation. Some patients may be candidates for thrombolysis or thrombectomy in ischaemic stroke, or neurosurgical evacuation of haematoma in intracranial bleeding. The outcome varies widely, reflecting the site and extent of cerebral damage.

Equally important are the non-structural, often reversible causes. Metabolic disturbances represent one of the most frequent categories. Hypoglycaemia is particularly important because it can cause irreversible neuronal injury if not corrected promptly, yet recovery can be immediate if glucose is given early. Hyperglycaemia, diabetic ketoacidosis, hepatic encephalopathy, and uraemia are also well-recognised culprits. Electrolyte imbalances, such as severe hyponatraemia or hypercalcaemia, can profoundly affect neuronal activity and consciousness. Identifying these disorders depends on rapid laboratory testing, and treatment is usually straightforward once the abnormality is recognised.

Drug intoxication and poisoning are another frequent cause of coma, especially in emergency settings. Opioid toxicity presents with miosis, respiratory depression, and reduced consciousness, and can be rapidly reversed with naloxone. Alcohol intoxication, benzodiazepines, and barbiturates are also common offenders. Environmental exposures such as carbon monoxide poisoning should not be overlooked, particularly when several individuals present with similar symptoms. Toxicology screening provides confirmation, but empiric antidotal therapy may be lifesaving before results are available.

From a clinical perspective, it is useful to distinguish between immediately reversible and non-reversible causes. Hypoglycaemia, opioid overdose, and some metabolic derangements can be corrected within minutes if recognised promptly. In contrast, massive strokes or severe traumatic injuries may not be reversible, but early identification is still vital to guide intervention, prognosis, and ongoing care.

Approaching the diagnostic process for coma in a structured and pragmatic manner is both clinically effective and cost-efficient. Time and resources can easily be wasted if rare causes are pursued too early, while common and reversible conditions remain overlooked. By beginning with simple, high-yield investigations – blood glucose, basic biochemistry, toxicology screens, and non-contrast CT – clinicians can often identify the diagnosis rapidly and institute treatment without delay. Advanced imaging, EEG, or invasive procedures should be reserved for patients in whom the cause remains unclear after first-line assessment.

This approach is not only economical but also life-saving. In many cases, a comatose patient may be restored to consciousness quickly if the underlying disorder is identified early. Administering intravenous glucose to a hypoglycaemic patient or naloxone to a suspected opioid overdose can be lifesaving and requires little more than clinical vigilance and basic resources. The principle of starting with the most common, treatable causes and working systematically towards the less frequent ones lies at the heart of good medical practice.

In daily clinical work, reversible causes such as metabolic disturbances, intoxication, and systemic infections account for a large proportion of coma presentations. Structural causes, particularly trauma and stroke, are also common and require urgent imaging to guide management. By integrating this pragmatic and structured approach into emergency care, healthcare professionals can improve diagnostic accuracy, reduce unnecessary investigations, and provide safe, effective, and timely treatment.

Ultimately, the goal is not only to save life but also to preserve neurological function and quality of life. Patient safety must remain paramount, and cost-effectiveness follows naturally when clinicians focus on common causes first, apply simple tests early, and reserve complex investigations for selected cases. This approach ensures that the management of coma is not only clinically sound but also efficient, sustainable, and aligned with the best principles of modern medical care. Always think of the common, reversible causes first.

Topic 27

Overdose and Loss of Capacity

Note to the reader: this case is more extensive than the others in this book. It has been deliberately expanded because it covers every important aspect of one of the most difficult situations a doctor can face: capacity, consent, teamwork across different agencies, and the application of the law. Its teaching value makes the extra detail essential.

The call from the ambulance service came late one afternoon. They were attending a 35-year-old woman who had taken a large overdose of paracetamol. She was distressed and refused to be taken to hospital. The paramedics knew the risk. In paracetamol poisoning, a patient may look well at first, but the drug silently damages the liver. Unless the antidote, intravenous N-acetylcysteine, is given within six to eight hours, the damage may become irreversible and fatal. The crew had tried to persuade her, but she refused. They contacted our practice for urgent help.

I was the on-call GP and reached the house within minutes. The atmosphere was tense. Marie, as I shall call her, was pacing up and down, her face red from tears, her voice angry and restless. She had discovered her husband's infidelity and in despair had swallowed the tablets. She told us that she did not care what happened to her and wanted to be left alone.

I sat with her and explained carefully that paracetamol poisoning is deceptive. Although she felt well, her liver was already under threat. In a few days she could become very ill, jaundiced, and confused, and she might die in great discomfort. Treatment was available and effective if started immediately. She listened briefly but dismissed my words. She repeated that nothing mattered.

It was clear she was not able to weigh the information. She could hear it but could not process or apply it to herself. The Mental Capacity Act 2005 (MCA) defines capacity as decision-specific and time-specific. A person must be able to understand, retain, and weigh the information relevant to the decision and communicate their choice. At that moment, Marie could not. Her overwhelming distress had robbed her of that ability.

The Act also says we must do everything possible to help a person decide before concluding they lack capacity. I tried again, speaking more slowly, breaking things down into simpler terms, and reminding her of her child who depended on her. But she rejected this, shaking her head. It was clear she lacked capacity for this decision.

Once that conclusion was reached, Section 5 of the Mental Capacity Act became crucial. Section 5 gives legal protection to healthcare professionals who provide care or treatment to someone who lacks capacity, provided two conditions are met: first, that they reasonably believe the person lacks capacity; and second, that they reasonably believe the act is in the person's best interests. This protection allows us to act lawfully when a patient is temporarily unable to make a safe decision. Without Section 5, intervening against her refusal might be considered assault. With Section 5, provided we act proportionately, we are protected.

Section 5 is not a licence for unlimited power. It requires that any action must be the least restrictive option available. That meant I could not simply order her to be taken by force. We had to attempt persuasion, involve the right support, and avoid restraint if possible.

At this point, accurate record-keeping became essential. I wrote down what she said, how she behaved, the explanations I gave, and the reasons I believed she lacked capacity. I noted the repeated attempts at persuasion and why they failed. I recorded that time was critical in paracetamol poisoning and why escalation was necessary. These records would not only support my judgment if later questioned but would also provide transparency for the crisis team, hospital staff, and psychiatric services.

I called the crisis team and requested police attendance. This was not done lightly, but it was necessary to make sure that treatment could be given safely. The crisis team arrived first. They spoke to her not about the tablets but about her pain. They listened, acknowledged her feelings, and reassured her that despair can pass. Their empathy softened the atmosphere.

The police arrived shortly after. They did not take over but stood quietly in the background. Their calm presence added authority without escalating the situation. They were ready to intervene if safety demanded it, but they allowed the healthcare professionals to lead.

The ambulance crew remained steady, prepared to transport her at any moment but showing patience and restraint.

After a long and difficult dialogue, with support from the crisis team and the quiet reassurance of the police, Marie finally agreed to hospital transfer. She was reluctant but consented voluntarily, and she walked to the ambulance without confrontation. I recorded carefully that she ultimately consented and that no restraint was used. This detail mattered: it showed that the least restrictive path had been achieved.

In hospital she was treated promptly with N-acetylcysteine. Blood tests confirmed the overdose was serious, but because treatment was given within the critical window her liver recovered. She also received psychiatric support for the crisis. Within days she stabilised and was discharged.

When she returned for follow-up, she was calmer and grateful. She admitted that at the time she could not think clearly or understand what was happening. She thanked us for acting when she could not. Seeing her restored to her usual self confirmed that the intervention was right.

Looking back, this case shows how the law, ethics, and teamwork come together in practice. Capacity is not fixed: even competent adults may lose it temporarily in a moment of overwhelming distress. Section 5 of the Mental Capacity Act is what allows us to act in such circumstances, but it also limits us: we must act in the patient's best interests, proportionately, and with the least restriction possible. Documentation is not a side issue;

it is the backbone of lawful and transparent practice. Every observation, every attempt at persuasion, and every step of reasoning must be recorded.

The case also underlined how essential teamwork is. The GP assessed capacity and coordinated decisions, the ambulance crew maintained readiness, the crisis team provided psychological expertise, and the police added authority and safety. Alone, none of us could have achieved a safe outcome. Together, we succeeded.

For junior doctors and GPs, the lesson is clear. In moments of crisis you may face the daunting task of overriding a patient's refusal. Do not be paralysed by fear of the law. Understand Section 5 of the Mental Capacity Act: if the patient cannot understand or weigh the information, and if your action is in their best interests, you are legally and ethically protected. Always record your reasoning in detail, involve colleagues, and choose the least restrictive option. Remember that you are not only protecting life in the moment but also safeguarding the patient's future autonomy. Intervention may feel uncomfortable at the time, but often patients look back with gratitude, recognising that these actions preserved their chance to live and decide again.

Topic 28

Weight Loss

Unexplained weight loss is a frequent presentation in general practice. Patients may notice their clothes becoming looser, relatives may raise concerns, or the change may be discovered incidentally during a consultation. It is often in general practice that the first assessment takes place, with hospital referral following later if necessary. Because the potential causes are many, a structured approach is essential to avoid both missed diagnoses and unnecessary investigation.

The first step is to establish whether the weight loss is voluntary or involuntary. Some people actively try to reduce their weight through dieting or exercise, while others may believe they have lost weight when in fact the scales show stability. Consistent measurement in the surgery, ideally with the same scales under similar conditions, ensures accuracy and avoids unnecessary alarm.

Once confirmed, the next question is whether the weight loss occurs with a preserved appetite or with reduced appetite. This simple distinction is extremely useful.

When appetite is preserved, the differential diagnosis is relatively narrow. The two classic causes are diabetes mellitus and thyrotoxicosis. In diabetes, patients may eat well yet continue to lose weight. They may also report thirst, frequent urination, fatigue, blurred vision, or dizziness. A random blood glucose or HbA1c usually confirms the diagnosis. In thyrotoxicosis, patients often describe weight loss despite a good appetite, together with sweating, heat intolerance, tremor, palpitations, or diarrhoea. Examination may reveal a goitre or tachycardia, and thyroid function tests provide confirmation. These two causes are common in general practice and should always be checked early.

When appetite is reduced, the possibilities are much wider. Gastrointestinal disease is one of the leading groups. Symptoms may arise from the mouth to the rectum: oral ulceration, dysphagia, peptic ulcer disease, or gastric carcinoma. Diarrhoea, bleeding, or abdominal pain may suggest Crohn's disease or ulcerative colitis. In the small bowel, malabsorption from coeliac disease or chronic pancreatitis is possible.

Colorectal disease is particularly important in the UK. Colorectal cancer is one of the most common malignancies presenting through weight loss, especially in older patients. It may cause iron deficiency anaemia, a change in bowel habit, rectal bleeding, or an abdominal mass.

Other systemic causes include endocrine disorders such as Addison's disease, where fatigue, hypotension, and pigmentation may accompany wasting.

Psychiatric illness is another common group. Depression often presents in primary care with anorexia, early morning waking, low mood, and loss of libido. Schizophrenia may lead to neglect, poor diet, or poverty. Anorexia nervosa, usually seen in young people, is marked by restrictive eating, amenorrhoea in women, and a distorted body image.

Malignancy is still the most feared diagnosis. Solid tumours of the lung, pancreas, stomach, or bowel may present late, with weight loss as the dominant feature. Haematological malignancies such as lymphoma, leukaemia, and multiple myeloma may present with lymphadenopathy, hepatosplenomegaly, night sweats, or bone pain. A crucial point is that malignancy is often detected late, particularly in disseminated or occult cancers, because early signs may be subtle or absent. For this reason, unexplained weight loss must always be taken seriously.

Chronic infection is another important category. Tuberculosis, though less common than in the past, is still seen, especially in immunocompromised patients. Chronic abscesses, subacute endocarditis, or bronchiectasis may also present with weight loss over weeks or months. Connective tissue and autoimmune diseases such as systemic lupus erythematosus, rheumatoid arthritis, polyarteritis nodosa, and dermatomyositis may also cause anorexia and wasting, often alongside systemic features like joint pain, pericarditis, or rash.

The rate of weight loss provides another important clue. Rapid loss over weeks or months is usually organic and serious, while slow loss over years may be linked to psychiatric, social, or chronic benign disease.

Examination should be thorough, but guided by the history. The thyroid may be enlarged or hypervascular in thyrotoxicosis. The cardiovascular system may reveal murmurs suggestive of endocarditis. The chest must be examined for clubbing, effusions, or lung masses. Abdominal palpation may detect hepatomegaly, splenomegaly, ascites, or masses. Lymph node enlargement may suggest lymphoma or leukaemia. Joints and skin should be examined for signs of autoimmune disease.

Investigations in primary care begin with simple tests. A full blood count may reveal anaemia, leukaemia, or myeloma, with iron deficiency anaemia being a classic red flag for colorectal cancer. ESR and CRP are useful markers of chronic inflammation, often raised in malignancy, myeloma, or infection. Renal and liver function tests may point to renal carcinoma, hepatoma, metastases, or abscess. Thyroid function tests and HbA1c will confirm or exclude the common endocrine causes. Serum protein electrophoresis may identify myeloma, while urinalysis can reveal haematuria or proteinuria.

Basic imaging is also valuable. A chest X-ray can show lung cancer, TB, or infection. Ultrasound may detect abdominal masses or organ enlargement. CT, MRI, endoscopy, and colonoscopy are generally arranged in secondary care once the initial work-up provides direction.

Although the potential causes are numerous, in everyday general practice most cases of unexplained weight loss can be traced back to a small number of conditions. The most frequent are malignancy, especially lung and bowel cancer; gastrointestinal disease, including malabsorption and inflammatory bowel disease; endocrine disorders, in particular diabetes and thyrotoxicosis; chronic infection, especially tuberculosis; and psychiatric illness, most commonly depression. These five categories should always be the first to consider, with rarer causes explored once the basics have been excluded.

A structured approach to weight loss does more than ensure diagnostic accuracy. It is also cost-effective and time-saving, because it narrows the focus to what matters most. Importantly, this efficiency is not at the expense of good care. On the contrary, a careful history and thorough examination often provide the strongest clues to the diagnosis, pointing the way forward before any tests are even ordered.

For junior doctors and GPs, the message is clear. Begin by confirming true weight loss, distinguish preserved from reduced appetite, consider the rate of loss, and keep the common serious causes firmly in mind. Remember that malignancy is often detected late, so vigilance is essential. Above all, never underestimate the value of history and examination – they remain the cornerstone of safe, effective, and compassionate practice.

Topic 29

Acute Abdomen

Note: this chapter is intentionally more extensive than the others, reflecting the breadth and importance of acute abdominal emergencies. The extended discussion is intended to give junior doctors and GPs a practical and structured approach to one of the most challenging presentations.

Acute abdomen is one of the most common and urgent clinical presentations in medicine. Many patients are first seen by their general practitioner, though most will be referred to Accident and Emergency (A&E) for assessment and management. The role of the GP is not always to make the final diagnosis, but to recognise the seriousness of the presentation, form a sensible differential diagnosis, and ensure rapid referral. Explaining to the patient what is suspected helps them understand the urgency, and it alerts hospital colleagues to the possible cause without delay.

Because the list of potential diagnoses is so extensive, a structured way of thinking is essential. The most practical approach is to begin with the anatomy. The abdomen can be divided into nine surface regions: right hypochondrium, epigastrium, left hypochondrium, right flank, umbilical region, left flank, right iliac fossa, suprapubic or hypogastric region, and left iliac fossa. Simply asking the patient to point to the site of their pain narrows the differential considerably. Some conditions, however, produce diffuse pain, as in a perforated viscus or peritonitis, and this must always be borne in mind.

Pain in the right hypochondrium usually reflects hepatobiliary disease. Biliary colic, acute cholecystitis, or ascending cholangitis are the leading causes, while hepatitis or liver abscess must also be considered. The presence of fever, jaundice, or rigors often helps to distinguish between these conditions. Epigastric pain is commonly due to peptic ulcer disease, gastritis, gastro-oesophageal reflux, or pancreatitis. A perforated ulcer typically causes sudden, severe pain that may radiate to the back. Associated nausea, vomiting, melaena, or haematemesis are important clues.

The left hypochondrium is most often affected by splenic pathology, such as rupture or infarction. Left-sided renal stones or pyelonephritis can also present with pain in this region. In the flanks, the most important structures are the kidneys and ureters. Renal colic is recognised by its colicky nature and radiation towards the groin or testicles in men, often accompanied by haematuria. Patients may also describe previous similar episodes. Other causes include urinary tract infection, renal abscess, or tumour.

Pain in the umbilical region may reflect disease of both small and large bowel. Intestinal obstruction, perforation, mesenteric ischaemia, Crohn's disease, ulcerative colitis, or an abdominal aortic aneurysm must all be considered. In children, intussusception is an additional possibility. The right iliac fossa is classically the site of acute appendicitis. Pain often begins centrally and only later localises as the peritoneum becomes irritated. Other causes include caecal carcinoma, Crohn's disease, or caecal tuberculosis. In women, ovarian or gynaecological disease can mimic appendicitis.

The suprapubic or hypogastric region may involve urinary or gynaecological pathology. In men, urinary retention, bladder infection, or pelvic abscess should be considered. In women, ectopic pregnancy, salpingitis, and ovarian torsion are vital to exclude. A pregnancy test is mandatory in any woman of reproductive age with lower abdominal pain. The left iliac fossa is the classical site of diverticulitis, particularly in older adults. Carcinoma of the sigmoid colon is another key cause, and perforation of diverticular disease may present dramatically with peritonitis.

Age can also refine the diagnosis. In children, appendicitis, mesenteric adenitis, and intussusception are common. In young adults, appendicitis dominates, along with biliary disease and, in women, gynaecological emergencies such as ectopic pregnancy or ovarian torsion. In the elderly, diverticulitis, bowel obstruction, a perforated viscus, and malignancy are the most frequent causes.

Once the anatomical location and likely causes are considered, examination should focus on the relevant area. Tenderness, guarding, and rebound suggest local peritoneal irritation. Palpable masses, hernias, organomegaly, or abdominal distension may provide additional clues. Investigations then support or confirm the provisional diagnosis. Blood tests are essential: a raised white cell count is typical in appendicitis, cholecystitis, or renal infection. Serum amylase (or lipase) supports pancreatitis. Abnormal liver function and bilirubin may indicate obstructive jaundice. Stool tests may reveal blood or mucus in colitis or carcinoma. Urinalysis is particularly valuable in renal or urinary causes, with haematuria a classic sign of renal colic. Blood cultures may be required if sepsis is suspected.

Imaging provides further clarity. A plain abdominal X-ray may show obstruction with air–fluid levels, or free air beneath the diaphragm in perforation. Ultrasound is excellent for gallstones, cholecystitis, gynaecological disease, and renal pathology. CT scanning has become central to the modern evaluation of the acute abdomen, clarifying obstruction, diverticulitis, perforation, or abscess. MRI is especially useful in pelvic disease. Endoscopy, including gastroscopy and colonoscopy, may be required when peptic ulcer disease or colorectal carcinoma are suspected.

In the UK, the five most common causes of acute abdomen are clearly established and should always remain at the front of the clinician's mind. Acute appendicitis remains the single most frequent surgical emergency, especially in younger patients. Biliary colic and acute cholecystitis are also highly prevalent, particularly in middle age, and together represent a large proportion of right upper quadrant presentations. Diverticulitis of the sigmoid colon is the dominant cause of left iliac fossa pain in older adults and may progress rapidly if perforation occurs. Bowel obstruction, whether arising from adhesions, hernia, or colorectal carcinoma, is another major and often life-threatening emergency. Finally, perforated peptic ulcer, though less common today thanks to the availability of proton pump inhibitors and Helicobacter pylori eradication, continues to present dramatically with sudden peritonitis. Collectively, these five conditions account for the majority of acute abdominal emergencies encountered in daily practice and must be actively considered in every assessment.

The acute abdomen requires rapid recognition, structured reasoning, and decisive referral. The most reliable method is to localise the pain, recall the anatomy of the region, consider the patient's age group, and then apply investigations to confirm the likely diagnosis. For GPs and junior doctors, the essential lesson is that careful history and examination almost always provide the strongest clue, while tests play a supporting role. A structured approach is both safe and efficient, ensuring that urgent cases are recognised and managed without delay. The strength of this method lies in its clarity and simplicity: observe carefully, think logically, and act decisively. Always return to anatomy as the starting point, for accurate localisation of pain combined with sound clinical assessment will guide the diagnosis more reliably than any investigation performed in isolation.

Topic 30

Epilepsy

Loss of consciousness is a common and often challenging presentation. It may arise from a simple faint or syncope, but occasionally represents an epileptic fit. The clinician's role is to determine whether the episode was a faint or a fit, to identify the possible cause, and to decide on the urgency of referral. This decision is crucial, as it guides whether immediate hospital admission or outpatient assessment is required. The distinction is not always straightforward, however, and demands careful clinical reasoning.

A detailed and focused history is the first essential step. Whether the patient is seen in hospital or in the community, it is vital to ask when and how the episode occurred. Fainting or syncope typically develops gradually, often with preceding dizziness, visual dimming, or a sense of warmth, allowing the patient to support themselves or sit down before falling. In contrast, an epileptic fit tends to occur suddenly and without warning; the patient may collapse abruptly and have no recollection of the event.

Clinical clues often assist in differentiation. In syncope, the patient may appear pale, sweaty, and bradycardic, recovering quickly once lying flat. There is usually no tongue biting, no urinary incontinence, and the return of consciousness is rapid. In epilepsy, tonic-clonic movements, tongue biting, and postictal confusion are characteristic. These simple observations, when interpreted carefully, often lead to the correct diagnosis.

Syncope itself may occur for various reasons. Vasovagal fainting, the most frequent type, can follow emotional stress, pain, fatigue, or standing for a long period in a hot environment. Micturition syncope is common when individuals, particularly men, rise suddenly from bed at night to pass urine without allowing time for the blood pressure to stabilise; the sudden postural change leads to venous pooling and a transient drop in cerebral blood flow. Orthostatic hypotension, dehydration, and certain antihypertensive drugs can produce a similar effect. In all these cases, the episode is brief, and recovery is spontaneous once the patient becomes supine.

Cardiac causes of syncope must always be kept in mind. Severe bradycardia, tachycardia exceeding 200 beats per minute, or other rhythm disturbances can markedly reduce cardiac output and brain perfusion. Complete heart block may lead to Stokes-Adams attacks, short episodes of collapse due to sudden failure of cardiac conduction. Once the ventricular rate stabilises around 30 beats per minute, symptoms usually subside, but if it drops below 20, recurrent attacks may occur. Ventricular tachycardia can also present with transient loss of consciousness. In these cases, pulse assessment and ECG recording confirm the diagnosis and guide further management.

Metabolic and biochemical disturbances can also mimic epilepsy. Hypoglycaemia is a well-recognised cause and may arise in diabetics who have taken excess insulin, missed a meal, or undertaken vigorous exercise, but it can also occur in non-diabetic individuals after prolonged fasting. Functional or reactive hypoglycaemia may follow a large carbohydrate meal, particularly in those who have had partial gastrectomy. Occasionally, recurrent hypoglycaemic attacks are due to an insulinoma, a benign pancreatic tumour producing excess insulin. Electrolyte disturbances such as hyponatraemia, hypernatraemia, or hypocalcaemia, as well as hepatic encephalopathy, may also result in fits or altered consciousness.

When fainting has been excluded, attention turns to epilepsy. The approach should begin by understanding the likely causes, then focusing the history and examination on those possibilities. Any initial investigations available in primary care - such as glucose, electrolytes, or ECG - can be arranged, but most patients will require referral to secondary care for further assessment and confirmation. A structured, stepwise approach ensures accuracy and avoids unnecessary delay.

Infective and inflammatory causes must be kept in mind. Meningitis, encephalitis, and cerebral abscess are important examples, and viral encephalitis may present with recurrent fits. Occasionally, malaria relapses with neurological symptoms. Autoimmune disorders such as systemic lupus erythematosus or autoimmune encephalitis are increasingly recognised as causes of seizures.

Other important causes of recurrent fits, particularly in older adults, include stroke – one of the leading causes in the elderly – and both primary and secondary brain tumours. Secondary deposits may arise from cancers of the breast, kidney, or bowel. Head injury, whether due to road traffic accidents or falls, is another significant cause. In some cases, despite thorough investigation, no cause is found; these are classified as idiopathic or cryptogenic epilepsy. Although the list of potential causes is long, concentrating on the common and age-related patterns makes the assessment practical and efficient.

Once epilepsy is suspected, assessment should proceed systematically. The patient's age provides a valuable guide. In children, congenital brain malformations, perinatal hypoxia, genetic conditions, and central nervous system infections are common. In adults, trauma, brain tumours, and cerebral abscesses predominate. In the elderly, cerebrovascular disease, degenerative changes, and secondary tumours are most frequent.

During history-taking, emphasis should be placed on identifying risk factors relevant to each age group. Ask about perinatal complications or family history in children; head injuries or previous infections in adults; and strokes, hypertension, or known malignancy in the elderly. This focused method avoids repetition, saves time, and directs the examination efficiently.

Physical examination must then be comprehensive and guided by the likely cause. Neck stiffness, fever, or focal neurological signs may suggest meningitis or abscess. Asymmetrical weakness or reflex changes can point to a localised lesion. Clubbing or chronic cough may indicate bronchial carcinoma with cerebral spread. The cardiovascular system should be examined for hypertension, murmurs, or atrial fibrillation, and the lungs for effusion, collapse, or tuberculosis. The abdomen should be checked for organomegaly or masses such as renal cell carcinoma, which can metastasise to the brain. These findings guide both diagnosis and urgency of referral.

Once the history and examination are complete, the clinician must decide which patients require immediate hospital admission and which can safely be investigated as outpatients. In general practice, syncope is usually benign and managed locally, whereas epilepsy demands specialist neurological evaluation. Warning features such as prolonged unconsciousness, postictal confusion, focal neurological signs, or recurrent attacks justify urgent referral.

In the United Kingdom, the most common causes of epilepsy vary by age group. In children, congenital brain injury and genetic disorders predominate; in adults, trauma and tumours are frequent; and in the elderly, stroke is by far the leading cause, followed by tumours and degenerative cerebral disease. Recognising these patterns enables efficient assessment and avoids unnecessary investigations.

The message is clear. When faced with transient loss of consciousness, begin by distinguishing between fainting and fits through a careful, critical history. Always consider the patient's age, as it provides key diagnostic clues. Concentrate on the common causes first - stroke, trauma, tumour, and infection - and refer promptly when epilepsy is suspected. This disciplined, logical approach saves time, prevents misdiagnosis, and ensures safe, effective, and compassionate patient care.

It is also worth emphasising that such a structured and selective approach is cost-effective and time-saving, yet never at the expense of quality or thoroughness. Good clinical judgement ensures that resources are used wisely, while maintaining the highest standards of patient care.

Comment

This discussion of the topic is intentionally more extensive than usual because it involves two interrelated presentations - fainting (syncope) and epilepsy. Understanding both together is essential to appreciate their differences and overlaps. It highlights how careful assessment, logical reasoning, and awareness of common causes enable the clinician to approach such cases with confidence and precision.

Topic 31

Haematemesis and Melaena

Haematemesis and melaena represent serious clinical emergencies which demand immediate attention and coordinated management, primarily within hospital settings. The general practitioner's role is usually limited to early recognition, initial resuscitation, and arranging urgent transfer to the emergency department. Prompt action - such as calling an ambulance and ensuring safe referral - often determines the outcome.

This condition may affect any age group, but it is particularly dangerous in patients over 50 years old. Mortality rises sharply among the elderly, who often have limited physiological reserve because of comorbidities such as COPD, heart disease, or diabetes. Their reduced ability to adapt to sudden circulatory collapse contributes to a poorer prognosis. In these emergencies, diagnostic work and treatment proceed simultaneously. Once the patient arrives, intravenous access is established immediately, fluids are started, and blood is taken for cross-matching. Early monitoring and stabilisation go hand in hand with the search for the underlying cause.

An important first step is confirming that the blood is of gastrointestinal origin. In children, swallowed blood from a nosebleed or pharyngeal injury can later be vomited, simulating haematemesis. Similarly, black stools do not always signify melaena; the tarry appearance may result from iron supplementation or medications containing bismuth. Awareness of such false positives prevents misinterpretation and unnecessary intervention.

Blood transfusion requires careful consideration, particularly in elderly patients with heart disease. Rapid transfusion can precipitate cardiac failure; hence blood should be infused slowly with close observation. In younger patients, tolerance is usually better, but anaemia or hypotension can still trigger myocardial ischaemia in those with pre-existing coronary disease. Vigilance is therefore essential.

In cases related to chronic liver disease, particularly cirrhosis, variceal bleeding presents a major hazard. Absorption of nitrogenous substances from the bowel may precipitate hepatic encephalopathy, while hypovolaemia can cause renal impairment or even acute renal failure. Severe bleeding may also impair retinal circulation and occasionally cause macular ischaemia. Thus, the effects of gastrointestinal bleeding often extend beyond the digestive tract, involving multiple organ systems.

The decision to transfuse blood is guided by both laboratory and clinical findings. A haemoglobin level below 10 g/dL, together with hypotension or tachycardia, usually justifies transfusion. However, each case should be judged individually, and early consultation with a surgeon or gastroenterologist is vital. Joint decision-making ensures appropriate timing of endoscopic or surgical intervention once the patient is stabilised.

When approaching diagnosis, it is vital to keep the process cost-effective and time-saving, yet never at the expense of patient care. This principle should guide every junior doctor's approach. Investigations must be chosen carefully and directed by the most probable causes, rather than ordered indiscriminately. Time lost on unnecessary tests can delay critical intervention and compromise patient safety.

In practical terms, the diagnostic reasoning should focus firmly on the four main causes of upper gastrointestinal bleeding: duodenal ulcer, gastric ulcer, gastric erosions, and oesophageal varices. These account for the majority of presentations encountered in clinical practice. Concentrating initially on these common pathologies allows prompt and rational investigation, early treatment, and efficient use of hospital resources. Rarer causes – such as coagulopathies, vascular malformations, or malignancies – should be considered only when these principal conditions are excluded by history, examination, or endoscopic findings.

A thoughtful, structured approach is a mark of clinical maturity. It saves time, reduces risk, and improves outcomes. Conversely, unfocused investigation reflects uncertainty and often wastes valuable time. Junior doctors must remember that effective diagnosis depends on reasoning, not on the quantity of tests ordered.

Standard packed-cell transfusions contain little or no clotting factors. Persistent or massive bleeding therefore calls for the use of fresh whole blood or fresh frozen plasma (FFP) and platelets to replace lost coagulation components. Neglecting this may result in continued bleeding despite adequate haemoglobin replacement.

The clinical history often provides the first and most important clues. Duodenal ulcer classically presents with intermittent epigastric pain, sometimes waking the patient at night and relieved by food or antacids. Gastric ulcer, by contrast, tends to cause pain soon after eating and may be associated with weight loss. Hiatus hernia and reflux disease are common in overweight patients who complain of burning retrosternal discomfort and regurgitation. Understanding these distinctions allows a focused and logical approach before investigations are undertaken.

Variceal bleeding is a separate and particularly severe category. It usually results from portal hypertension secondary to cirrhosis caused by chronic hepatitis, alcohol misuse, or biliary disease. Portal obstruction may also occur from old umbilical sepsis, hepatocellular carcinoma, pancreatic cancer, or portal vein thrombosis associated with polycythaemia. Occasionally, portal pyaemia following an intra-abdominal infection such as an appendiceal abscess can be responsible.

Clinical features of portal hypertension include hepatosplenomegaly, ascites, dilated abdominal veins, spider naevi, palmar erythema, and sometimes a flapping tremor from hepatic encephalopathy. In advanced disease, the patient may exhibit lower-limb oedema or pulmonary congestion, reflecting systemic circulatory compromise.

Examination in the emergency department has two aims: first, to assess the degree of blood loss, and second, to look for clues to the source of bleeding. Assessment focuses on the patient's level of consciousness, pulse rate, blood pressure, temperature, and peripheral perfusion. Pallor, sweating, tachycardia, and hypotension suggest significant loss. Examination for liver disease, abdominal tenderness, or cachexia helps narrow the diagnostic direction.

Investigations are guided by the patient's stability. Once resuscitated, upper gastrointestinal endoscopy becomes the investigation of choice, allowing both diagnosis and treatment through injection therapy, banding, or cauterisation. When endoscopy is not feasible, a barium study may be used later, though it is less sensitive and should never be attempted during active bleeding. Endoscopy remains the cornerstone for both confirming the cause and controlling the haemorrhage.

In every major gastrointestinal bleed, early cooperation between medical and surgical teams is essential. The physician's role focuses on resuscitation, stabilisation, and medical management, including endoscopic therapy and correction of coagulopathy. The surgical team must be involved from the outset, as emergency intervention may be required if endoscopic control fails or the patient deteriorates. Effective communication between both departments ensures continuity of care and significantly improves survival outcomes.

Haematemesis and melaena should always be regarded as manifestations of an underlying pathology, rather than diseases in their own right. Management begins with stabilisation - airway protection, intravenous fluids, and blood replacement - followed by identification and treatment of the source. The ultimate goal is to prevent recurrence by addressing the precipitating factor, whether that be eradication of H. pylori, withdrawal of ulcerogenic medication, or control of portal hypertension.

Summary

Haematemesis and melaena are dramatic and potentially fatal emergencies. For the general practitioner, recognition and rapid referral are the key responsibilities. For junior doctors, the essential skill lies in disciplined, clinically guided reasoning - focusing first on duodenal ulcer, gastric ulcer, gastric erosions, and oesophageal varices as the principal causes. The diagnostic approach must be cost-effective and time-saving, but never careless or superficial. Each step should add value to patient care. Early resuscitation, multidisciplinary coordination, and close cooperation between medical and surgical teams remain the foundation of safe, efficient, and life-saving practice.

Topic 32

Dysphagia

Note: The complexity of this topic requires a broader discussion than usual, to cover the main categories and clinical reasoning involved.

Dysphagia, or difficulty in swallowing, is a not uncommon symptom in general practice. While general practitioners may encounter occasional cases, most patients are referred to hospital or specialist clinics for assessment. Such centres often receive referrals from a wide area, as dysphagia may reflect a neurological, structural, or malignant disorder requiring multidisciplinary input. Nevertheless, it is a topic worth revising in primary care, since an alert GP can often recognise early warning signs and refer promptly, saving valuable time and preventing diagnostic delay.

A psychogenic cause is often the first consideration, particularly in younger or middle-aged women. The complaint is usually of an inability to swallow rather than pain or obstruction, often triggered by emotional stress and accompanied by anxiety features such as tremor, sweating, and palpitations. Examination and investigations are typically normal, and reassurance is usually sufficient once organic disease has been excluded.

Another rare but classical cause is Sjögren's syndrome, encountered mainly by rheumatologists. The presentation includes dryness of the eyes and mouth due to autoimmune destruction of lacrimal and salivary glands, producing difficulty in chewing and swallowing. The tongue appears red and tender, the lips cracked, and the salivary glands may be enlarged. Associated features include arthritis, lymphadenopathy, hepatosplenomegaly, neuropathy, and Raynaud's phenomenon.

Inflammatory or neoplastic lesions in the mouth are usually obvious on inspection. Ulcers, leukoplakia, or carcinoma of the tongue, tonsil, or pharynx produce painful dysphagia. Glossitis associated with iron-deficiency anaemia and acute infections such as pharyngitis, peritonsillar abscess, or tonsillitis may temporarily interfere with swallowing but are self-limiting. Mechanical obstruction by a foreign body, such as a fishbone, is occasionally seen but easily identified and managed.

Neuromuscular disorders form another important group, often referred to as bulbar dysphagia. This results from failure of the swallowing muscles due to neurological disease. Historically important causes such as diphtheria and poliomyelitis are now rare in the United Kingdom. Today, the problem is more often seen in motor neurone disease, myasthenia gravis, or other degenerative brainstem disorders. The difficulty lies in initiating swallowing; once the bolus reaches the pharynx, food may regurgitate through the nose or enter the larynx, leading to coughing and choking.

A pharyngeal pouch (Zenker's diverticulum) occurs mainly in elderly people and represents a herniation of mucosa through a weak point in the upper oesophageal wall. Food and liquid may regurgitate immediately after swallowing or when the patient bends forward. Gurgling in the neck during drinking and recurrent aspiration pneumonia are typical findings.

Another uncommon but significant condition is sideropenic dysphagia (Plummer-Vinson syndrome) resulting from long-standing iron deficiency. Thin mucosal webs form in the upper oesophagus, causing solids – but not liquids – to stick immediately after swallowing. Glossitis and angular cheilitis are frequent companions. The condition progresses slowly and may lead to chronic narrowing if untreated.

Mechanical obstruction may arise anywhere along the oesophagus. If a delay occurs between swallowing and the sensation of food sticking, the obstruction is usually in the lower part. External compression from mediastinal lymphadenopathy, aortic aneurysm, or an aberrant subclavian artery may occasionally produce similar symptoms. Systemic sclerosis can also involve the oesophagus, producing late-stage fibrosis, aperistalsis, and reflux.

Achalasia is another major cause of dysphagia, due to degeneration of the myenteric (Auerbach's) plexus. The condition progresses insidiously and may lead to a markedly dilated, 'mega-oesophagus.' Patients experience difficulty with both solids and liquids, sometimes accompanied by chest pain or nocturnal regurgitation of undigested food, occasionally causing aspiration.

Benign oesophageal strictures are almost always secondary to chronic reflux oesophagitis, frequently associated with a sliding hiatus hernia. Repeated acid exposure results in scarring and narrowing near the lower end, producing dysphagia that begins with solids.

Carcinoma of the oesophagus remains the most serious diagnosis. It develops silently until the tumour encroaches on the lumen, leading to progressive difficulty with solids and later liquids. Early on, patients may note discomfort at the start of a meal that settles after a few mouthfuls. Unlike achalasia, dysphagia in malignancy is progressive rather than intermittent. Radiological imaging may reveal irregular narrowing and loss of peristalsis, but endoscopy with biopsy provides definitive diagnosis.

In the United Kingdom, four causes account for most presentations of dysphagia. The commonest is stroke or cerebrovascular disease, where neurological injury to the medulla or higher swallowing centres prevents normal initiation of swallowing. The second is oesophageal carcinoma with malignant stricture. The third is gastro-oesophageal reflux disease (GORD) leading to peptic oesophagitis and benign stricturing. The fourth is achalasia or other oesophageal motility disorders, where failure of relaxation of the lower oesophageal sphincter (LOS) impedes the passage of both solids and liquids. Together, these four conditions represent the majority of cases seen across UK practice.

When assessing dysphagia, it is practical to follow an anatomical and functional sequence. The history should clarify whether the problem involves solids, liquids, or both; whether it is intermittent or progressive;

and whether pain, regurgitation, or aspiration accompany swallowing. The presence of dryness of the mouth, iron-deficiency anaemia, or neurological symptoms provides additional clues to the underlying cause.

Examination should be targeted and confirmatory, rather than repetitive. Inspect the mouth and pharynx for ulcers, infection, or tumour, palpate the neck for lymph nodes or masses, and assess cranial nerve function if a neurological cause is suspected. Chest examination may reveal evidence of aspiration or mediastinal disease.

Investigations include blood tests for anaemia or autoimmune markers, a barium swallow to outline structural abnormalities, and endoscopy for direct visualisation and biopsy. CT scanning of the neck and chest is used to detect extrinsic compression, local invasion, or mediastinal lymphadenopathy, while MRI is valuable for soft-tissue or brainstem involvement. In malignancy, both imaging methods assist in staging and surgical planning. These modalities complement but never replace careful clinical assessment and endoscopy. In complex or suspected malignant cases, multidisciplinary input involving radiology, gastroenterology, and surgery is essential for optimal management.

Comment

Although dysphagia may arise from many different conditions, the clinician's first responsibility is to focus on the most probable and clinically significant causes. For doctors in primary care or junior hospital posts, constructing an initial diagnostic block based on the four common UK causes ensures an organised, safe, and cost-effective assessment. Once these have been confirmed or excluded, attention can then shift to rarer or complex disorders. The guiding rule is simple: think of the common causes first, reason systematically, and never sacrifice thoroughness or patient safety for speed. This balanced approach consistently achieves both efficiency and high-quality care.

Author Biography

Dr Omar J Hassouna
General Practitioner, Medical Author, Former Chair of Local GPs
With nearly five decades of experience working within the National Health Service (NHS), Dr Hassouna has devoted his professional life to clinical medicine, medical leadership, and education. His medical career began in London in 1976 with a clinical attachment, after which he undertook a wide range of hospital posts that laid the foundation for a broad and practical understanding of medicine.

Diverse Medical Experience
Dr Hassouna's early hospital work included paediatrics, geriatric acute medicine in Wales, and psychiatry, where he developed a strong appreciation of mental health conditions such as anxiety, depression, and psychosis. As a medical registrar, he gained further experience in diabetes, haematology, respiratory medicine, cardiology, and gastroenterology, managing both acute and chronic medical conditions. He also spent time in gynaecology and obstetrics, further widening my clinical exposure and reinforcing the importance of holistic patient care.

These formative years shaped his diagnostic thinking and clinical judgement, skills that later became central themes in his medical writing.

Transition to General Practice
In 1983, Dr Hassouna transitioned into general practice, initially joining a training practice before becoming a partner in 1984. This move required a

significant shift from hospital-based medicine to managing undifferentiated presentations in the community. Over time, he established and led several dedicated clinics, including antenatal, postnatal, hypertension, diabetes, respiratory (COPD and asthma), thyroid, and gout clinics. These services enabled comprehensive and continuity-based care tailored to community needs.

He also established a WHO-recognised Travel Clinic, providing risk assessment, travel advice, vaccinations including yellow fever, and official certification. This service supported both local patients and travellers from further afield.

Leadership and Administrative Roles

From 2007 to 2010, Dr Hassouna served as Chair of the local GPs. During this period, he attended monthly Primary Care Trust (PCT) meetings and chaired numerous GP forums. This role provided first-hand insight into the interface between frontline general practice and healthcare policy. It strengthened his understanding of system pressures, governance, and the practical challenges faced by clinicians working within evolving NHS structures.

Out-of-Hours and Urgent Care Experience

Throughout the 1980s and 1990s, Dr Hassouna worked extensively in out-of-hours services. This was an era before mobile phones, electronic records, or centralised triage systems, often requiring long journeys and rapid decision-making under difficult conditions. These experiences were instrumental in developing clinical resilience, independence, and pragmatic problem-solving skills.

Following 2000, he also worked within Urgent Care Centres, adapting to newer models of emergency and unscheduled care and witnessing first-hand the increasing pressures on acute services.

Forensic and Social Medicine

Alongside general practice, Dr Hassouna served as a Police Surgeon, working closely with law enforcement on cases involving drug misuse, assault, sexual offences, and deaths in custody. This role demanded meticulous clinical assessment, legal awareness, and close collaboration with police and courts.

He also worked with social services, assessing patients for disability and mobility allowances. Conducting home visits provided invaluable insight into the social determinants of health and reinforced the importance of contextual medicine beyond clinical settings.

Continuing Professional Development

Dr Hassouna remains committed to lifelong learning, obtaining postgraduate diplomas in Dermatology (Cardiff University) and Diabetes Care (Warwick University). These qualifications strengthened his specialist input within primary care and informed both his clinical and educational work.

Qualifications

MBCHB, Baghdad
LMSSA, London
Practical Dermatology Diploma, Cardiff University
Diploma in Diabetes Care, Warwick University

Authorship and Educational Contribution

Drawing on decades of real-world clinical experience, the author has published three medical books, each with a distinct but complementary focus:

Challenging Scenarios in Medicine (2025)

This book presents complex and often high-risk clinical situations encountered in general practice, accident and emergency departments, hospital wards, and community settings. It focuses on safe decision-making, uncertainty, and practical management in challenging circumstances.

Real-World Challenges in Clinical Medicine (2026)

Building on the first book, this volume places greater emphasis on everyday clinical dilemmas faced by GPs and junior doctors, particularly in under-resourced and time-pressured environments. It highlights diagnostic pitfalls, communication challenges, premature discharges, and situations where clinicians are left managing risk with limited support.

Practical Approaches to Clinical Diagnosis (2026)

This book adopts a topic-based, structured approach to diagnosis. It is designed to help clinicians reach accurate diagnoses efficiently by focusing on common presentations, pattern recognition, and clinically relevant reasoning. The aim is to save time, reduce unnecessary investigations, control costs, and enhance patient safety.

Together, these books reflect a progression from complex scenarios, to real-world pressures, to practical diagnostic frameworks.

A note from the Author

Over the decades, I have witnessed profound changes in the NHS, particularly since 2005. Increasing workload, workforce shortages, population growth, ageing demographics, resource limitations, and administrative inefficiencies have placed the system under sustained strain. Staff morale has declined, and patient presentations have become more complex. These realities provided strong motivation for translating clinical experience into educational resources for the next generation of clinicians.

My professional journey reflects a sustained commitment to patient care, medical education, and mentorship. Through my clinical work, leadership roles, and writing, I aim to support medical students, junior doctors, and general practitioners in navigating the increasing complexity of modern medicine and maintaining high standards of safe, thoughtful clinical practice.

Dr Omar Hassouna

Notes

Notes